Radical Leisure

How Mothers Gain Well-Being and Control through Participation in Exercise Classes

---

Janet L. Currie, PhD

Radical Leisure

How Mothers Gain Well-Being and Control through Participation in Exercise Classes

---

Janet L. Currie, PhD

COMMON GROUND RESEARCH NETWORKS 2018

First published in 2018
as part of the Health, Wellness & Society Book Imprint
doi: 10.18848/978-1-86335-015-0/CGP (Full Book)

Common Ground Research Networks
2001 South First Street, Suite 202
University of Illinois Research Park
Champaign, IL
61820

Library of Congress Cataloging-in-Publication Data

Names: Currie, Janet L., author.
Title: Radical leisure : how mothers gain well-being and control through
    participation in exercise classes / Janet L. Currie, PhD.
Description: Champaign, IL : Common Ground Research Networks, 2018. |
    Includes bibliographical references and index.
Identifiers: LCCN 2017059777 (print) | LCCN 2018023373 (ebook) | ISBN
    9781863350211 (pdf) | ISBN 9781863350150 (hardback : alk. paper) | ISBN
    9781863350167 (paperback : alk. paper)
Subjects: LCSH: Exercise for women. | Women--Health and hygiene. | Leisure.
Classification: LCC GV482 (ebook) | LCC GV482 .C87 2018 (print) | DDC
    613.7/1082--dc23
LC record available at https://lccn.loc.gov/2017059777

Cover Photo Credit: Phillip Kalantzis-Cope

Table of Contents

CHAPTER 1

At Your Leisure: The Importance of Healthy, Active Leisure for Mothers

WORKING MOTHERS, MENTAL HEALTH, LEISURE AND LIFESTYLE

Psychological distress is a major health issue for women across their lifespan (ADHA, 2005; Steel et al., 2013, p. 9). Nearly half of all Australians will experience a mental health disorder at some point in their lifetime; however, this is likely to affect more women than men (ADHA, 2005; ABS, 2008). Depression and anxiety are the most commonly experienced mental health disorders (Slade et al., 2009; Beggs et al., 2007). For example, a recent survey of more than 10,000 Australian women found that over 40 per cent have been professionally diagnosed with depression or anxiety (Brown, Abbott, Pirotta, & Camilleri, 2017).

The highest prevalence of mental health conditions in Australia exists among young women. Further, analyses of recent Australian National Mental Health and Well-Being Surveys identified anxiety disorders as an ever-increasing problem facing middle-aged women (ABS, 2008; Holden et al., 2013; Slade, 2009). As mothers in Australia continue to experience high levels of stress, policy-makers have called for programs and action to address the issue (Reavely et al., 2011).

With almost one in three Australian mothers reporting depressive symptoms at least once during her child's first four years (Woolhouse, Gartland, Mensah, & Brown, 2014), they commonly experience tiredness and emotional stress (APS, 2015). The social and psychological factors causing tiredness include the vicious circle of tension at home, guilt and anxiety about working outside the home, and a lack of involvement in social or community life outside work and home. In the dreadful rush and crush as mothers endure these stressful circumstances and attempt to cope under excessive workloads, some also:

- hold themselves and others to extremely high standards (e.g. with housework)

- exhibit low self-esteem and the need to earn the approval of others,

- put other people's needs constantly before their own, and then

- feel resentment at doing this, then guilt about the resentment they feel.

Mothers do not always recognise their "off" button, or feel justified in pressing it to take time out from their daily routine. They often feel reluctant to delegate household tasks. Many are habituated to staying at home, in and around any outside paid employment. The majority only feel justified in taking any leisure time when household duties have been satisfactorily completed (Patty, 2016). Unfortunately, an average of six in ten Australian mothers do not meet the recommended 2.5 hours of weekly physical activity because they report feeling "too tired" or consider it "too hard" to find the time (Brown et al., 2017).

Individual feelings of despair, anger and grief can be related not only to a woman's experience, but also to her oppression within society. Isolation, lack of support, low self-esteem, lack of leisure or personal freedom are indicative of living within patriarchy. Stress levels can continue to mount once paid work is completed, since domestic work and childcare responsibilities fall disproportionately on women (Losoncz, 2011). Women working at home can also feel added stress from the mundane nature and drudgery of household tasks. Due to the "invisible" nature of housework and the fact that housewives do not get paid, they feel undervalued within the household and community.

Throughout this book, the term "working mothers" refers to women who carry out paid and/or unpaid work, and who are also mothers. This is to reflect the valid nature of work conducted in the home, and the fact that women wish to have their legitimate efforts recognised by society. All mothers work; however, for ease of reference, paid work will be noted as "employment" or "outside" work.

Mental health includes having a positive self-esteem, general feeling of coping with daily tasks, and a sense of balance in our social and emotional well-being. It's important for mothers to be able to access coping strategies for stress management and a greater sense of well-being (beyondblue, 2016).

RADICAL LEISURE: THE POWER OF LEISURE TO CREATE A SPACE OF ONE'S OWN

This idea of the enclosure of the individual (mother) in space (home and family) underpins Foucault's (1977) theory of disciplinary technology. According to Foucault, power includes the whole range of disciplinary technologies such as rules, norms, checks, and surveillance, which control, transform, and condition an individual. An essential part of power includes control of space through limits, prohibitions, or obligations. Power acts over the body and over society through the smallest elements, such as the family, and through gender relations. It is not an instrument of oppression, but rather a strategy for training the body (Patton, 1979).

Discourse is an idiosyncratic way of talking about a discipline. It includes the accepted rules, statements, ways of understanding and processes: a body of knowledge (Foucault, 1977). Perceptions of "truth" are produced in and by discourses, and discourse is often created through processes of normalisation. Subjugated knowledges or hidden, alternative ideas, theories and points of view are usually discredited by "experts," or not spoken about, treated as taboo subjects. Postnatal depression was one such area not openly discussed even twenty years ago.

Due to destigmatisation, acknowledgement and greater social acceptance of the issue, mothers have been able to more readily seek assistance and feel that they're not alone (Gellhorn, 2016; NSWCC, 1994; Swan, 2006).

However, mothers do feel social pressure to conform and cope. Extremes do not fit in. We must speak the "truth," or in the case of the ideal mother, gain social acceptance and approval, through always being selflessly available and putting others' needs ahead of her own:

> Power never ceases its interrogation, its inquisition, its regulation of truth: it institutionalizes, professionalizes, and rewards its pursuit (Foucault, 1976, p. 93).

"Normal" or "good" mothers are meant to adhere as closely as possible to the ideology of motherhood. They are meant to be happy and coping at all times (NSWCC, 1994). This involves a normative standard of a socially constructed role of someone who devotes her personal time, energy, and resources to attending to the needs and welfare of her children and family. It is therefore not surprising that lack of leisure, lack of time to self and poor mental health are major concerns often expressed by working mothers (Gjerdingen et al., 2000).

However, wherever there is power there is the possibility for resistance, or the uprising of knowledges previously discredited (Foucault, 1987). In this situation, dominant discourses are under constant challenge by individuals who struggle at the conscious or bodily level to create new identities, meanings, and subject positions for themselves. Resistance to the dominant discourse at the level of the individual subject is the first stage in the production of alternative forms of knowledge or, where such alternatives already exist, of winning individuals over to these discourses and gradually increasing their social power (Weedon, 1987).

Using Foucault's (1977) poststructuralist notions of the concepts of power, discourse and resistance, this book suggests that exercise classes taken at a mother's leisure offer her an outlet to challenge some aspects of her subordination. The act of taking "time out" to exercise when they please is radical as it challenges the ideology of motherhood, or the emphasis of the mother's care for others (Wearing, 1990). It creates a new space that can be reserved just for the leisure of the mother herself.

Leisure is a quality experience, where the nature of the activity is characterised by perceived freedom (Henderson, Bialeschki, Shaw, & Freysinger 1989). A space for one's leisure may take the form of a mental space, such as daydreaming during the vacuuming; a time space, such as having a rest in a comfy chair, putting all of the chores on hold; or an activity space, where activities such as walking, coffee with friends or exercise classes may be pursued. Gaining personal space for leisure is defined as:

> space physical or metaphorical over which one has control to fill with whatever persons, objects, activities or thoughts that one chooses. There are many possibilities here (Wearing, 1998, p. 149).

According to the personal accounts of a group of mothers I interviewed, exercise classes can provide one avenue for mothers to find such a space, and take more control over their own health and lifestyle. Exercise classes may be classified as leisure if the mother is intrinsically motivated to take part and senses personal freedom during the activity (Henderson et al., 1989).

In this book, "exercise classes" refer to aerobics or group exercise classes to music of about sixty minutes' duration, commonly found in local gyms, community centres and fitness clubs. The mothers surveyed for this book engaged in weekly classes for at least three months, with each session consisting of a warmup, followed by low-impact (no running or jumping) freestyle moves or aerobics, muscle conditioning exercises for the whole body, a cool-down, stretch, and relax. The venue or hall did not contain mirrors and it was a non-commercial, supportive atmosphere, with childcare available.

CONCLUSION

Feminist writers have adopted some of Foucault's ideas on discourse and subjectivity; however, they argue for women to be conceptualised as active, creative subjects rather than passive recipients of structural forces or constraining discourse (Smith, 1988; Weedon, 1987). In this way, the individual with her/his mind or body can actively resist alignments of power with a dynamism not seen as possible by Foucault (1977). Throughout this book, value is placed on the individual perspectives that women have provided me regarding their own leisure experiences. If leisure is defined as being an experience, then we may greater understand and be able to interpret mothers' thoughts, feelings and responses by speaking with participants, and authentically reporting those experiences in their own words. This book goes some way to making the mothers' little-known experiences of exercise class participation visible and understood. In writing it, I acknowledge the oppression and inequalities that exist in their health and leisure opportunities.

Finally, this book suggests that exercise classes for leisure offer women an outlet to challenge some aspects of their subordination. The act of a mother taking 'time out' to exercise when she pleases may be considered radical as it challenges the dominant discourse of motherhood. It creates a new space taken *at one's leisure*, able to be reserved just for the mother herself.

Mental health benefits await mothers who are able to create active leisure space for themselves. The next chapter outlines the nature of stress that may be typically experienced by mothers. It also contains an analysis of how this stress can manifest, and how it can detract from feelings of subjective wellness.

CHAPTER 2

Why Are Mothers Stressed?

INTRODUCTION

According to a major Health Survey of 10,377 Australian women aged 18 to 89 years, approximately 40 per cent have been professionally diagnosed with depression or anxiety. Those aged eighteen to thirty-five years are the most anxious age group among women in Australia, experiencing "mild" levels of anxiety, with the authors blaming the new age of social media, being "ever-ready" to be on Instagram and the constant checking of phones. Nearly half of the women surveyed reported that on several days a week they:

- worry excessively about different things

- become easily annoyed or distracted

- have trouble sleeping (Brown et al., 2017, p. 3).

Despite rates of women's paid employment increasing, women have not compensated by reducing the quantity of work they complete around the home. According to the ABS (2009), employed women working full-time spend almost 65 hours in a combination of paid work and household work (total work). However, an online survey of 1,009 mothers conducted by the Research Unit for a major Australian health and pharmaceutical company found employed women work on average up to eighty hours a week in paid employment and running their household (Patty, 2016).

Women remain overwhelmingly responsible for child-rearing and domestic chores (ABS, 2012a), and this is reflected in their overall health. While men are spending slightly more time on traditionally "female" domestic activities such as cooking and laundry than in 1992, most mothers still retain primary responsibility for family care and domestic matters, spending almost twice as much time on housework and childcare than men, even when they increase their time in paid employment (ABS, 2009; Baxter, 2013; de Vaus, 2009; Hochschild, 1989). Employed women with children are more likely than other women or any other group for that matter to feel rushed or pressed for time, with 62 per cent always or often being rushed, 32 per cent experiencing this state sometimes, and only 6 per cent experiencing it rarely or never (Baxter, 2013). In conclusion, Baxter (2013, p. 7) noted:

It is valuable to be reminded of the need to find the balance between these competing demands on our time, and to be mindful of finding time to care for our own well-being as well as that of others around us.

As a mother attempts to fulfil multiple roles in the home, community, and workplace as if each were full-time, she risks her mental health (ADHA, 2005). Employed mothers often just expand their usual household and personal responsibilities around their paid work involvement. Through not reallocating some of their traditional tasks, dual-career wives often feel stressed from the juggling involved in meeting the demands of husband, children, home, school, family, community, friends, and career (APS, 2015). Due to mothers retaining overall responsibility for childcare, the conflict between the parenting, career and any other responsible roles often produces immense stress (Botkin, 1989).

For example, mothers coping with multiple role responsibilities say they experience the following problems:

- childcare problems associated with working outside the home

- feelings of guilt about involvement in outside work and not remaining at home

- no time for self

- fatigue and tiredness after work

- no help from other family members with overwhelming household responsibilities (APS, 2015; Lee, 2001; Pearce, 1989).

Most mothers say they feel stressed and overwhelmed, going regularly for weeks without even a single minute relaxing on their own (Hitchcock, 2009). They feel they live their lives entirely for other people, or state that chores are not shared equally between themselves and their partners, or that their current domestic arrangement is unfair. When quizzed on their domestic workloads it emerges that most mothers take on the bulk of home chores, and more than half said they do not have time for their own hobbies or interests. Mothers in one study said they obtained an average of 17 minutes of "me time" to themselves each day, due to packed schedules managing children, work, and chores (Schulte, 2014). Unfortunately, due to these pressures, women focus on their children and family's health and happiness first and, as a result, most commonly overlook their own needs (Patty, 2016):

There is a lot of pressure for mums to 'keep up appearances,' whether it's juggling a career with motherhood, or keeping the household running smoothly. Unsurprisingly, guilt plays a big part in this.

HOW MOTHERS KNOW THEY ARE STRESSED

Stress is the non-specific response of the body to any demand upon it (Seyle, 1974). Stress, in this instance, can also be defined as the emotional and physical reaction to the pressures that society places upon mothers to conform and live up to expectations. The majority of mothers surveyed for this book say they do suffer from stress. They know they're feeling stressed when they detect individual symptoms like headaches. Some mothers revealed they experience physical symptoms such as "heart palpitations and tightness of throat":

- I get headaches and asthma when under stress.

- I get headaches and feel cranky.

- I often find it hard to cope with a nine-month-old baby and a husband that works twelve hours a day. Often, I get very frustrated and exhausted muscle tension, tired, headaches.

- Looking after three children, I get headaches.

For Lorraine, a 31-year-old with two young children, stress means, "Everyday life, being a mother trying to get everything done and mainly getting irritable and tired."

Role Overload as a Cause of Stress

Stressors are the individual stress-producing factors which elicit the stress response (Seyle, 1974). The constant demands of cleaning the house, shopping for and feeding the family, caring for children plus completing any outside paid work or additional caring and community obligations may produce tension, stress and fatigue in a mother.

When mothers were aware of feeling stressed, they described the stressors as situations related to attempting to complete multiple roles:

- Yes, when trying to juggle two children, part-time work and getting household tasks done etc.

- My 3½ year old son driving me "up the wall" at times. Mainly due to jealousy of new baby plus money worries at present [are also] causing family stress.

- Feeling there is not enough time in the day to do everything. i.e. Spending time with the children, housework, work in my studio, etc. etc.

- Recovering from almost "burn-out" after several years in social welfare work.

- [Feeling] dependent on family/work.

Julie, a 41-year-old mother of three teenage children, says she suffers from stress when one member of the family is sick or if the responsibilities of her busy job become overwhelming to her.

Role overload and proliferation is a type of role pressure or stressor particularly relevant to married women who simultaneously perform the roles of wife, mother, and employee, each with its own competing set of demands (Schulte, 2014). The factors influencing a woman's perception of her multiple-role situation as stressful include:

1. traditionalism of her own sex role norms;

2. the influence of any role reinforcers, and

3. the woman's perception of herself as a success or failure in her roles (Woods, 1980).

If a mother feels ultimately responsible for the overall success of the home, in terms of fulfilling a range of tasks. This can include caring, cooking and cleaning, and also feeling responsible for the happiness of others, including children, so it can lead to high levels of stress. Stress has a major effect on the health of women who are careers or involved in multiple roles such as domestic work, unpaid caring and paid employment.

Typical descriptions given by mothers indicating these kinds of pressure situations, which lead to feelings of stress, include:

- Coping with my husband's retrenchment, unemployment. Loss of loved ones and a very busy life, lots of running around.

- Worrying about my elderly mother who has Parkinson's disease and is living on her own; Christmas corning up, children's happiness.

- Christmas coming. Children at home for the holidays and entertainment for them.

- Just the general running of the household with two children. Husband has been working long hours. Juggling finances, getting ready for Christmas, e.g. shopping.

- New baby, difficult toddler, a stressed-out husband who expects a lot from me, financial stress, and Christmas.

- Extremely busy life, full-time work with a lot of responsibility and commitment with three children and their schools, and helping look after an elderly mother; frantic weekends.

Due to the fact that women juggle so many tasks and fulfil so many roles, they often have little time left for themselves:

- I try and cram too many activities in my day and I just do not have enough time for everything. Too little time, too much to do.

- Little children jumping all over me with not a minute's peace.

The Detrimental Effect of This Lifestyle on Mental Health

The distress or negative stress experienced by women in attempting to be in control and cope with the motherhood role has been known to contribute to anxiety states (Spielberger, 1989). Add to this any financial, relationship, or health difficulties, and the mother certainly has a lot to deal with. This was confirmed in recent surveys of Australian women's health (Grace Papers, 2016; Patty, 2016).

> Mums are putting themselves second to their family needs and suffering for it. With only one in 20 working mums taking the necessary time for rest and recuperation, as well as working 80 hours a week, it's no wonder they are feeling overwhelmed, stressed, and fatigued. And this ill health, both physically and mentally, is likely to affect their family dynamics and their children's overall well-being. Working mums are constantly told to strive for balance and to make time for themselves. And while many mums are responsible for taking on too great a burden and putting themselves last, external constraints also play a huge role in hindering them from taking proper care of themselves. Career demands, time pressures, technological advances blurring the lines between work and home, childcare constraints, the tightening of paid parental leave, gender inequality; it all contributes to the stress and over-reliance placed on mums (Grace Papers, 2016).

Amy is an example of a mother experiencing role overload and proliferation. She completes extra work for her husband's company in addition to her own home tasks. She also expressed a desire to get fit and "into shape" once again after the recent birth of her baby son. She told me how the feeling of "no time left for herself" increased her stress levels and was detrimental to her mental well-being.

Her house was very neat and tidy. Piles of neatly folded nappies and washing lay in an ironing room. She appeared organised and in control; however, it came at a cost a constant feeling of expecting herself to complete a set schedule of jobs, and be constantly on the go. Only when she felt all of her self-designated tasks were finished did she feel justified in exercising or taking any time out:

Janet: Does anything stress you?

Amy: Oh yes! My four-year-old son. And looking after the baby just turned nine months.

Janet: How do you feel if you are stressed?

Amy: Just uptight and worrying about getting everything done that I want to get done, so that I can feel relaxed in myself.

Janet: Do you feel that it's expected of you?

Amy: I expect it of myself. Because I've got to have things done, I've got to be organised, that's just the way I am. But my husband does expect a lot of me.

Julie is another typical example of an extremely busy wife, mother, worker, counsellor, cook, cleaner, career, and part-time "father." She expresses guilt if she is not constantly on the go and feels conditioned to be that way. She finds that her leisure has to be fast-paced so she does not feel like she's "doing nothing," or being lazy. She even classifies herself as "superwoman":

> I'd say so, yes. To the point I've got such a busy life and if I sit down at home for five minutes and do nothing, I feel really guilty that I am not on the go. I do not get a lot of time to myself, but when I do, um, I have got such a busy life, I find it hard to stop and do nothing.

Mothers tend to place high expectations on themselves. The mothers who spoke with me expressed a real sense of obligation to first complete all household chores, with every task completed to a very high standard, before even contemplating taking a break. The effort and emotional energy involved in caring for children can also limit women's leisure options and create stress by making mothers feel constrained by a limited sense of freedom. For example, Sue had not been able to exercise for years due to her work obligations, care of children and busy life at home, restricting her sense of freedom:

> With the children, I had them all very close together, so they were all in nappies or whatever, and this is the first year they've been at school, so I'm free to do whatever I want to do.

Merron claimed to be in a similar situation:

> It's something I have not done since I had Deanne. You know, to have half a day away from the kids. I love them, but to not have any family around, you know, to sort of have a break from the kids, a day or a half-day to do whatever I want to do, that would be nice. We've never been out since we had the kids, and Chrissie's nearly six. We've never been to dinner or away from them or anything like that. They go everywhere we go.

Merron also revealed to me that her philosophy or ethic of care about being a mum was so strong, she "would not pawn her kids out" to childcare. She also liked to be organised and feel "on top of things" all the time.

The reasons for mothers experiencing high stress levels are many; however, they are often related to the ethic of care associated with "good" mothering (Currie, 2009). Societal norms are for women to be devoted fully to their role in their career and to be totally effective at maintaining an efficient and hygienic household. As a consequence, women are often reluctant to delegate tasks, and sacrifice themselves before choosing to take time out. Mothers are deluged with media images of confident, proud, nurturing, attractive mothers who capably prepare gourmet meals and entertain the children, as well as being a loving wife all after a day of outside work. The ethics of care surrounding being a good mother means women (a) find it difficult to feel entitled to take time out for daily leisure, (b) if they overcome the constraints, find it difficult or inconvenient to access options, and (c) if they do, often feel guilty as a consequence, or are worried about the unattended household chores mounting up in the background.

This lack of leisure time and access to physical activity is to the detriment of women's mental, social, and physical health. As participation in leisure activities strongly associates with health and well-being (ABS, 2012b; Payne, 2010), it is essential that we as a society help improve women's access to it. To help manage stress, it is recommended that individual mothers:

1. understand how they experience stress

2. identify the stressors that cause stress

3. are aware of their current stress management techniques and understand whether they're healthy or unhealthy

4. find ways to manage stress (APA, 2011).

"SOMETHING'S GOTTA GIVE": EXERCISE FOR A MOTHER'S WELL-BEING

According to the World Health Organization (WHO, 2009) and the AGDH (2014), physical inactivity is the fourth leading cause of death due to non-communicable disease such as heart disease, stroke, diabetes, and cancers worldwide, contributing to over three million preventable deaths annually (6 per cent of deaths globally). Physical inactivity is also estimated to be:

- the main cause for approximately 21-25 per cent of breast and colon cancers, 27 per cent of diabetes and approximately 30 per cent of the ischemic heart disease burden.

- the second greatest contributor, behind tobacco smoking, to the cancer burden in Australia.

Nearly 70 per cent of Australian adults are either sedentary or have low levels of physical activity that is, are not completing the recommended thirty minutes of moderate intensity physical activity per day (AGDH, 2014). Women have lower rates of participation in physical activity than men in Australia (ABS, 2013a, 2013b, 2012c). Alarmingly, levels of physical activity tend to dramatically decline as we age. The World Health Organization (2016) believes the overall trend in individuals living in Westernised nations toward general lifestyle sedentariness, or high levels of physical inactivity, to be due in part to insufficient participation in physical active pastimes during leisure time (recognised globally as participating in less than 30 minutes of moderate intensity physical activity on most days of the week), and to an increase in sedentary behaviours as part of the activities undertaken at work and at home (AGDH, 2014).

Inactive people miss out on the significant individual health benefits to be gained from regular participation in sport and physical recreation. Engaging in regular physical activity—even of moderate intensity—can reduce the risk of developing a range of adverse medical conditions, including cardiovascular disease, colon and breast cancers, Type 2 diabetes, osteoporosis, obesity, and injury (Blair, Kohl, & Barlow, 1993). Being physically active can also assist in managing stress, depression, and anxiety, and in enhancing mental alertness (Biddle, 1995; Biddle, Fox, & Boutcher, 2000). Increasing physical activity levels for females is essential for improving health and mental well-being (Bull et al., 2004). Currently, walking is cited as the most popular form of physical activity for women, followed by gym and fitness, however, participation rates have been decreasing across all groups in recent years (ABS, 2015).

CONCLUSION

There is obviously a lack of fitness activities that can appeal to and readily cater for busy working mothers. If mothers recognise the value of active leisure as positively helping them manage stress and cope with a busy lifestyle, then we may see greater numbers taking part. Exercise participation has long been validated as associated with reduced anxiety levels, decreased depression and improved mood (Anderson & Sivakumar, 2013; Cramer, Nieman, & Lee, 1991; van Minnen, Hendriks, & Olff, 2010). The next chapter explains the underlying mechanisms which mediate the exercise–stress reduction relationship (Clow & Edmonds, 2014; Lam & Riba, 2016; Wankel & Berger, 1991) and can help to improve a mother's quality of life.

CHAPTER 3

Exercise as Stress Management

THE CONCEPT OF LEISURE AS A "THERAPEUTIC HEALTH EXPERIENCE"

Leisure may be conceptualised as an "experience." It is a period of time or activity during which an individual has a relative freedom of choice to do whatever they choose. It is often described as the free time we have remaining after we have completed all work, chores, and other obligations. The key feature that it is freely chosen allows us to experience a sense of control over our lives.

Leisure is characterised by:

- freedom of choice

- enjoyment

- relaxation

- intrinsic motivation and lack of evaluation

- sense of involvement

- a desire to separate or escape from the everyday routine world.

The personal satisfaction gained from leisure participation (Csikszentmihalyi, 1975; Csikszentmihalyi & Csikszentmihalyi, 1988; Csikszentmihalyi & Kleiber, 1991; Hamilton-Smith & Driscoll, 1990) results in enhancement of mood state (Hull, 1991; Hamilton-Smith, 1992). Therefore, the perceived quality of the leisure experience is paramount, as that personal rating directly affects and equates to the personal benefits accrued to the participant (Biddle & Mutrie, 2007; Wankel, 1992).

Leisure has been found to significantly increase one's resilience to stress and to improve mental and physical health (De Benedette, 1988; Iwasaki, Mannell, Smale, & Butcher 2005; Rosato, 1990). Exercise for leisure has been used as an effective mode of therapy for illnesses ranging from phobias to anxiety and depression, and for stress management (Sachs, 1982; Taylor, Sallis, & Needle, 1985). It has been recommended as having a potential therapeutic role for the treatment of pain, alcoholism, anxiety, bulimia, hypertension, addiction, depression, and anorexia nervosa (Biddle & Mutrie, 2007). In fact, results of clinical studies suggest that acute physical activity, noncultic meditation and a quiet rest session can all be equally effective in reducing state anxiety (Bahrke & Morgan, 1978; Paluska & Schwenk, 2000). Regular exercise is able to significantly decrease depressive symptoms in people experiencing depression. Anxiety symptoms and panic disorder also improve significantly with regular exercise (Paluska & Schwenk, 2000).

THE BENEFITS TO MOOD AND SENSE OF MENTAL WELL-BEING ASSOCIATED WITH EXERCISE PARTICIPATION

The related research literature has been able to widely document a range of evidence-based psychological benefits or mood enhancements associated with exercise participation including:

- release of pent-up emotional tension

- creative problem solving during the exercise session

- enhanced self-esteem

- greater sense of competence and internal control over events

- greater mental clarity after exercise

- less anxiety

- less depression

- mood stabilisation

- fun, play, joy (Cox, 2012; Paluska & Schwenk, 2000; Taylor, Sallis, & Needle, 1985).

Regular exercise alleviates negative mood states such as depression and anxiety (Byrne & Byrne, 1993; Dorinsky, 1984; Labbe, Welsh, & Delaney, 1988; Paluska & Schwenk, 2000). Beneficial effects appear to equal those of meditation or relaxation. For example, taking part in aerobic or strength training such as a running program has been able to produce consistently positive mood enhancement, with significant decreases in tension, confusion, fatigue, anxiety, depression, and anger, while maintaining high levels of vigour all of which is representative of positive mental health (Weinberg, Jackson, & Kolodny, 1988). However, these benefits can occur for even less vigorous or intense forms of exercise, where participants do not even have to improve fitness levels throughout the program (Bahrke & Morgan, 1978; Berger & Owen; 1989; Young, 1979). That is, the exercise does not need to be overly intense or "aerobic" in nature (Berger & Owen, 1989).

This is in sync with national physical activity campaigns advocating that people do not need to become serious sportspeople, but rather that physical activity should be undertaken regularly and simply perceived as an enjoyable part of everyday life. Most importantly for mothers, simple forms of low-intensity exercise, such as walking or low-impact exercise classes, may help in dealing with daily stressors (Currie, 2004; Morgan, 1979; Weinberg, Jackson, & Kolodny, 1988).

EXERCISE HELPS MOTHERS COPE WITH STRESS

Exercise participation is associated with less tension, less anxiety, less anger, and less fatigue that is, a generally improved mood state (Farrell, Gates, Maksud, & Morgan 1982). Conversely, regular exercisers have claimed to experience increased nervousness if prevented from exercising (Carmack & Martens, 1979). Various studies analysing self-reported measures of decreased state anxiety following engagement in acute physical activity have concluded that exercise caused tension reduction (Bahrke & Morgan, 1978; Dienstbier et al., 1981; Morgan, 1979; Morgan et al., 1980). As blood plasma levels of ß-endorphin have been reported to increase with exercise, especially running (Farrell, 1985; Goldfarb, Hatfield, Sforzo, & Flynn 1987; Grossman & Sutton 1985; Steinberg & Sykes, 1985), this has been proposed as the underlying mechanism for inhibiting extreme reactions to stress or pain and so improving coping ability (Steinberg & Sykes, 1985).

In a related study, 61 stressed, employed women were randomly assigned to either aerobic exercise (walking/jogging) or progressive relaxation interventions. The participants included chronically stressed, sedentary employed women recruited from the community (aged 24 to 59 years, average 40 years). They were screened to meet the following criteria:

1. Experienced effects from at least two persistent work-related stressors.

2. Scored 5 or above on Walk's (1956) Tension Thermometer.

3. Exercised less than three times per week for less than thirty minutes over the past three months.

4. Willing to be randomly assigned to either aerobic or progressive relaxation groups.

5. Employed for more than twelve hours per week.

Thirty-one subjects were assigned to exercise and 30 to relaxation, meeting once a week for one and a half hours over an eight-week program. Complete pre-test data was obtained from 50, due to lack of attendance at the first session. At the fourteen-month follow-up, 39 of the 50 were located, and it was found that 18 remained in the exercise group, 21 with relaxation. Both intervention groups reported significantly less anxiety and greater self-efficacy. In addition, subjects tended to increase their use of problem-focused coping as compared with emotion-focused coping. As a result of the physical activity, subjects felt less tense, more aware of how stress affected them and in greater individual control (Long & Haney, 1988b). This may be due somewhat to greater awareness of the feeling of relaxation, knowledge of how to access that, and self-efficacy in having a "coping strategy" available.

In a program of relatively shorter duration, 29 employees who participated in an 18-week employee aerobic fitness class program stated that they felt the classes helped them in various ways, the largest effect being subjective stress reduction, followed by increased stamina/endurance, improvement in mood and improvement in self-concept. Fitness or aerobic classes were held twice per week and took place right after work in a worksite conference room. It is interesting to note that all subjects volunteered for the study and 82 per cent were women (Imm, 1990).

People engaging in regular exercise are less vulnerable to the adverse effects of life stress than those who are less fit (Brown, 1991). Part of the reason for the improvements in well-being may be due to "self-selection" that is, happier and less stressed individuals tend to opt in to healthier lifestyles and also exercise more often (de Geus, van Doomen, & Orlebeke 1993; Long, 1983; Schafer, 1987). However, the good news is that exercise can be used as a prophylaxis against stress for fit or unfit individuals (Long, 1983; Roth, 1989). Participation in exercise per se, and not just achievement of increased fitness levels, can reduce self-reported stress.

Participation in individual activities such as walking, cycling, aerobics, jogging, swimming, and weight training offers people a certain amount of flexibility and freedom that might not exist if they were playing a team sport, such as tennis or netball. Some activities can be completed alone, outdoors or indoors, at flexible times, regardless of weather conditions. That being said, there has been little research including group exercise or aerobics classes as the exercise mode or intervention, and whether mothers feel it is acceptable to them and believe it increases states of subjective well-being. This is despite gym and fitness classes being the second most popular recreational activity for Australian women (ABS, 2015).

EXPLANATIONS FOR THE EXERCISE–STRESS REDUCTION RELATIONSHIP

The Endorphin Hypothesis

"Endorphin" is a term used to indicate any substance that exhibits opiate characteristics when subjected to clinical tests (Rosato, 1990). Essentially, this means that endorphins belong to the same family of drugs as those such as opioid analgesics or heroin. Participation in physical activity such as running can lead to powerful changes in emotional states (Allen, 1990; Harber & Sutton, 1984; Morgan, 1985), even producing the psychological adaptation called the "runner's high" (Pargman & Baker, 1980). As endorphins are released during exercise (Black, Chesher, & Starmer 1979; Farrell, 1985; Haier, Quaid, & Mills 1981; Kelly, 1986), the proposed linkage between exercise, endorphins, and pain reduction has led to the belief that exercise participation induces an analgesic state within an individual

(Farrell, 1985; Kelly, 1986; Padawer & Levine, 1992). Research has been able to demonstrate that exercise increases the level of endogenous opioid activity in the central and peripheral nervous system, leading to these analgesic effects (Harber & Sutton, 1984; Morgan, 1985).

Some studies have shown that when opioid antagonists have been administered in individuals following regular exercise, the endorphin-produced analgesic effects were able to be attenuated, but there were no concomitant changes in the mental health benefits to an individual, suggesting that an exercise-related surge in endorphins may not completely account for mental health benefits in many studies (Carr et al., 1981). Markoff, Ryan, & Young's (1982) study also refuted the hypothesis that endorphins serve as the biochemical basis for the runner's high. Mood changes studied before and after a 10-mile (16-kilometre) run did not reverse with or without naloxone (an endorphin antagonist) treatment, suggesting that mood elevations were not endorphin-mediated. Inconsistent results may be due to the different doses of naloxone administered in the experiments (Harber & Sutton, 1984), the different kinds of exercise or intensity prescribed (Steinberg & Sykes, 1985), or the subjects involved. However, as previously mentioned, running can lead to powerful changes in emotional states (Allen, 1990; Harber & Sutton, 1984; Morgan, 1985) and there is strong evidence available to demonstrate that exercise and regular activity positively impact the pathophysiological processes of anxiety (Anderson & Sivakumar, 2013).

Physiological Exertion and Tension Release

A physiological explanation for the reduction in anxiety from participation in acute exercise stems from the fact that physical exertion is a natural usage and consumption of physiological arousal and tension. Exercise has the ability to partially exhaust an individual and inhibit their capacity for further arousal (Anshel, 2006; Driscoll, 1976). In other words, it can use up energy that might otherwise have been spent on negative outcomes of stress, such as anxiety. The individual feels less tense after exercising, experiences less muscle tension and feels more relaxed overall.

Confidence and Control

The psychological benefits of developing a better-looking body or feeling more comfortable or confident with one's self as a result of exercising can enhance self-esteem and self-image. This makes us naturally "feel good." Any awareness during the exercise experience of it being an uplifting activity can improve our mood (Lazarus, 1980). If a mother can gain an "uplift" or "flow state" (Csikszentmihalyi, 1975) as part of a leisure experience, this may ease the burden of busy or monotonous work schedules.

Another explanation for the exercise–mental health phenomenon is the increased internal locus of control or individual sense of perceived control and mastery over one's own situation gained from regular physical exercise (Simons et al., 1985). A sense of control over one's environment is important because the belief that one can control events has been shown to reduce stress responsivity (Brown, 1991).

Time Out

An important theory explaining the reduced anxiety possible after acute exercise is the time out or distraction theory proposed by Bahrke and Morgan (1978). Brown (1991) called this concept "attentional focus," whereby the engagement in exercise turned people's attention away, even if only momentarily, from negative stress:

> By providing a temporary respite from life stress, exercise may serve a beneficial restorative function that allows people to deal with stressful circumstances more effectively (Brown, 1991, p. 560).

Psychological mechanisms such as distraction and mastery may mediate the reductions in anxiety scores (Martinson, Hoffart, & Solberg, 1989). De Benedette (1988) combined distraction theory with the proposed channelling of negative energy:

> The act of exercising itself may help to reduce stress. Exercise replaces the ambiguous aspect of psychosocial stress with concrete physical stress. It also acts as a distraction from stress and channels repressed anger and frustration into physical activities (De Benedette, 1988, p. 193).

Holidays as Time Out

Davidson (1992) argued that holidays make a significant contribution to the well-being of mothers. Holidays can assist with relaxation and mental recovery from everyday routines. The women in Davidson's (1992, p. 108) sample conceptualised holidays as being:

> a time away from their normal place of work, their home, with either a reduced workload or an increase in opportunities to do what they want.

Holidays are a way for women to slow down and escape for a while from their normally hectic lives. They are a popular leisure pastime during which women are able to disrupt normal routines, and interrupt the domination of clock time and work routines (Deem, 1986). The break from the normal routine may allow for feelings of relaxation, rejuvenation and revival.

Exercise as a Time Out Strategy for Busy Working Mothers

Through exercise, women can access time out from their busy schedules. Engaging in exercise classes could be thought of as having the benefits of a brief holiday. It is time where the normal workload can be reduced for example, if accessing childcare and gives women a break from the normal routine. When mothers take the time to exercise as part of their leisure, their stress levels diminish and well-being increases. Betsy Wearing similarly discovered:

There is no doubt in my mind, as in the mind of respondents, that those mothers who made a concerted effect to carve out leisure for themselves, gained in terms of time and space just for themselves and also in terms of their self-esteem, general sense of well-being, ability to control their situation of unpaid labour in the home and the stresses involved in child-care (Wearing, 1990, p. 54).

Leisure in the form of space and time out leads to greater well-being in women, possibly through feeling greater control of their situation in power relationships (Currie, 2004; Wearing, 1990).

CONCLUSION

Women, especially as mothers, face real barriers to accessing leisure, including lack of time, money, and childcare. Unless these immediate barriers are easily overcome, women would not feel encouraged to be involved in sport or leisure if it will interfere with their perceived primary role as carer for spouse, children, family, and home. A mother, through self-imposed standards measured against society's ethic of care, experiences feelings of guilt, and might not feel willing to involve herself in exercise for leisure. This is to the detriment of her health and well-being. These attitudinal barriers need to be broken down, and leisure facilities have to become more user-friendly if we are to increase women's access to leisure. This might include offering childcare (pm as well as am) within centres and activities on worksites, plus making a range of affordable, safe, sociable and varied activities available for women in the community.

This underlines the importance for mothers of establishing both spatial and temporal markers separating work from play—"a room of one's own"—to find time for herself (Lenskyj, 1988). Additional access to leisure opportunities can enhance our quality of life (Driver, Brown, & Peterson, 1991). For women, leisure is one social sphere which inspires positive potential for self-development and resistance to the definitions of "wife," "mother," "supporter," and "carer" (Wearing & Wearing, 1990).

Research evidence suggests that mood states such as anxiety can be modified by exercise (Abood, 1984; Anthony, 1991; Berger, 1984a; Choi et al., 1993; Frazier & Nagy, 1989; Leith & Taylor, 1990; Paluska & Schwenk, 2000). Yoga, progressive relaxation, and exercise may assist mothers in decreasing their levels of anxiety and stress (Long & Haney, 1988a; Berger & Owen, 1989; Martinson et al., 1989). However, exercise which involves aerobic or muscle conditioning is associated with greater health benefits, including an improved body shape and toning of muscles (Berger, 1984b; De Benedette, 1988; Pearce, 1993). Women may also feel greater energy, body tone and condition, which may engender further improvements to mood.

The next chapter provides a background to the body image of women. As the physical, mental, social and spiritual aspects of individual health are interrelated, and since we move our bodies during exercise, it is important to understand this issue, because it can positively or negatively affect anxiety reduction and the exercise experience.

CHAPTER 4

Women, Exercise, and the Search for the Perfect Body

INTRODUCTION

When women gain physical fitness, they reap mental health rewards such as experiencing improvements in mood, less anxiety and depression, and feeling more positive about their appearance (Brownell, 1991; O'Dea, 1992; Weiss, 1979; WHO/FIMS Committee on Physical Activity for Health, 1995). However, the ideal body shape often aimed for is lean and physically fit in appearance (Biddulph, Elliot, Faldt, Fowler, & Dugdale, 1984; Brownell, 1991; Davis, 1990; Pearce, 1993; Schulze, 1990; van Gyn, Randolph, & Bell 1989; Wilfley, Grilo, & Brownell 1994). The perceived benefits of having this slim, taut, youthful and athletic body drive many women to engage in excessive exercise and dietary behaviour (Duquin, 1989; Kenen, 1987; Paxton et al., 1991; Pearce, 1993; Redican & Hadley, 1988; Wilfley et al., 1994).

There are many exercise regimes and dietary programs today offering total body transformations: "The ideal fit feminine body is an ever-elusive goal" (Markula & Pringle, 2006, p. 163). However, the body is not so plastic that it can be shaped at will. We all have our own individual genetic and biological determinations that limit the amount of change possible (Bouchard & Johnson, 1988; Wilfley et al., 1994). If women fool themselves into believing that their body is infinitely malleable and can be shaped using diet and/or an exercise program to achieve the socially constructed aesthetic ideal, they will most likely experience great frustration and stress (Wilfley et al., 1994, p. 45). True empowerment is only possible when we have naturally moved towards our own goals of optimising our personal body shape, tone and physical condition, and we feel satisfied and accept the outcome. This chapter explores women's body image, pursuit of societal ideals, and body image as an incentive to exercise.

BODY IMAGE

Body image refers to an individual's perception of her/his own body (Treble, Blacklock, & McCormack 1990, p. 76). It includes:

> surface, depth, and postural pictures of the body as well as the attitudes, emotions, and personality reactions of individuals towards their bodies (Kolb, 1959 in van Gyn, Randolph, & Bell 1989, p. 466).

An individual's perception of her body shape or appearance can be positive or negative, realistic or unrealistic, and can be contributed to by personal experiences and other people's attitudes, reactions or comments (Ben-Tovim, 1992; Hart, Leary, & Rejeski 1989; Saltman, 1991; Vargas, 2015). The most common and obvious attitude held by virtually all women is "feeling fat," whether they actually are or not according to national height for weight charts (Ben-Tovim, 1992, p. 12).

A woman's level of dissatisfaction with her own body shape increases according to her proportionate increase in size above the standard norm or average shape for women in society (Davis, 1985; Howson, 2004). Further, the women participating in Davis's (1985) study who were most satisfied with their body shape were those with the tallest, most slender bodies those closest to the societal ideal. Women express greater negative concerns with their body image more frequently than men, and body image has a greater effect on women's self-esteem than on men's (Cooke, 1994; Chernin, 1993; Davis, 1990; Huon et al., 1990; Saltman, 1991; Tiggemann & Pennington, 1990; van Gyn et al., 1989).

Unfortunately, many women hold a distorted personal body image (Perutz, 1970; Sanford, 1984). This means a woman's perception of her own shape may be different to her actual body structure and appearance her body image lacks realism or accuracy. The degree of satisfaction with various body parts can affect or distort total body image. For example, a study conducted by Tucker (1985) discovered that women believed they were too large in their thighs, hips and waist. The lower half of their body caused the greatest dissatisfaction and they tended to base their overall body image on this factor. Men tend to base or rate their overall body image on the perception of their upper body chest, shoulders, and arms (Tucker, 1985).

A woman's perception of her own appearance and state of health affects her body image (Kelson, Kearney-Cooke, & Lansky 1990; Vargas, 2015). Body image is higher for those women who feel that their body is functioning healthily. This has implications for the benefits of regular exercise. Not only can it regulate a wide range of physiological processes, it can in turn positively impact body image (WHO/FIMS Committee on Physical Activity for Health, 1995). Physical activity participation in general has an overall positive impact on personal body image (Anshell, 2006; Biddle, 1991; O'Dea, 2007). Exercising helps us to consider what we feel like on the inside and to enjoy the movement rather than being concerned with what we look like from the outside.

Dissatisfaction with one's body shape appears to have become almost a cultural norm for women, referred to as 'normative discontent' by Imm and Pruitt (1991, p. 94). For example, of the 274 girls who answered a questionnaire by Biddulph et al. (1984, p. 34), 172 or 63 per cent wanted to lose weight. Treble, Blacklock, & McCormack (1990, p. 76) researched the alarming fact that some 34 per cent of women who were not overweight still wished to reduce their weight anyhow. The preference of body shape among the women in van Gyn et al.'s study (1989) was for a figure with shoulders and hips of similar width. Silberstein, Stiegel-Moore, Timko, & Rodin (1988, p. 224) tested women on their perceived ideal body shape/figure. Seventy-five per cent of the females chose an ideal figure that was thinner than their own perceived figure. Twice as many women (26.7 per cent) as men (12.8 per cent) selected an ideal that was two or more figures apart from their own perceived figure on the Body Size Drawing continuum.

The women participating in a study by Kelson et al. (1990) who focused the most on external body parts such as thighs, breasts and nose were the group most worried about their appearance in public and receiving negative appraisals from others. These women reported wearing cosmetics more often to attract attention away from any body part that they were self-conscious about. With make-up only a temporary camouflage, it will not have any lasting impact on the underlying overall body image.

Women with the most dissatisfied body image can be those assessing parts of their body that deviate most from the societal ideal, such as a flat chest or obese stomach. The greatest dissatisfaction expressed by women in van Gyn et al.'s (1989, p. 466) study was with the size of the:

- hips (71 per cent)

- buttocks (60 per cent) and

- abdomen (59 per cent).

According to medical authorities, 70 per cent of Australian girls and women are on a "serious diet" (Williamson, 1981, p. 19). Corresponding with the preoccupation with dieting among adolescent schoolgirls is a widespread dissatisfaction with the body and consequent desire to alter its image (Huon, 1992, p. 19). This condition may only increase as the levels of overweight and obesity increase in society.

The prevalence of women's body image dissatisfaction appears to be a global issue; it has been at consistently high levels for many decades. The large-scale research conducted by Dove (2016) included one-on-one interviews with 10,500 females across thirteen countries (6,000 women aged 18 to 64 and 4,500 girls aged 10 to 17 years in thirteen countries: India, the U.S., the U.K., Brazil, China, Japan, Turkey, Canada, Germany, Russia, Mexico, South Africa, Australia), revealing that women's confidence in their bodies is on a steady decline, with:

> low body esteem becoming a unifying challenge shared by women and girls around the world regardless of age or geography.

Women in Australia were categorised by the Dove (2016) researchers as 'Modernists,' wanting to "be it all and have it all," but then feeling immense pressure in an attempt to look beautiful and seemingly achieve this. Ironically, Australian women are acutely aware of the pressures they experience in wishing to achieve 'the look,' but commonly exhibit concurrent low levels of self-esteem. Sadly, as girls and women grow older, the pressure they feel to retain beauty increases while their own individual body confidence level decreases (Dove, 2017).

The negative impact of low body esteem on a woman's lifestyle included over 8 in 10 women (85 per cent) saying they would opt out of important life activities such as trying out for a team or club, going to the beach, or engaging with family or loved ones, when they do not feel good about the way they look (Dove, 2016). Feeling uneasy about one's own body can lead to restrictions in choice of clothes or participation in certain activities which expose disliked body parts (Smith, 1995). Chernin (1981, p. 25) revealed stories about women's preoccupation with their body weight, and their dislike of, and uneasiness with, their bodies, or certain parts:

> Many would grab their skin and squeeze it as we talked, with the grimace of distaste language cannot translate into itself.

Our body image is a function of the experiences that we have had, the physical activities we have engaged in and the lifestyle we expose our bodies to, as well as our degree of self-esteem and acceptance. It is potentially open to change in the future. It is important, therefore, that our social experiences, including partaking in classes at fitness clubs, are positive and our mental health is resilient. The next section discusses the relationship between body image, desired body shapes and mental health.

BODY IMAGE AND MENTAL HEALTH

Physical appearance and attractiveness are important aspects of self-concept in women (Kelson et al., 1990; Saltman, 1991; Salusso-Deonier & Schwarzkopf, 1991, Vargas, 2015). Females perceive great advantages in being slim (Paxton et al., 1991; Travis, 1988). They associate a high degree of thinness with:

- a popular personality

- good-looking appearance

- intelligence

- achievement (Chernin, 1993; Paxton, 1991; Wolf, 1994).

However, these are only perceptions. There is no research evidence available to date which confirms that women who are thin are happier than those women who are less thin.

Five hundred and twelve subjects in a study by Tiggemann and Rothblum (1985) rated their perceptions when viewing images of fat and thin people. Fat people were rated as less happy and less attractive than thin people. Images of average-weight people were not supplied as a comparison. Paxton et al. (1991) conducted a study on adolescent boys' and girls' perceptions on thin-ness. Females perceived thinness as being more of an advantage to them in real-life situations compared with males. For instance:

- 88 per cent of females stated that they would be happier if they were thin

- 90 per cent said they would be more successful

- 81 per cent said it would indicate how good-looking they were

- 80 per cent stated that it would indicate how many friends they would have and 'dates' they would attain

- 89 per cent believed that it would suggest how intelligent they were, and

- 93 per cent thought that it would be an indication of how easily they would achieve what they want.

An ideal female body shape characterised by sleek, slender lines tends to symbolise to other women a high degree of self-control, hard work and success (Barsky, 1988; Brownell, 1991; Glassner, 1988). Imperfections such as overweight can be viewed as symptoms of laziness or even moral failure (Barsky, 1988; Brownell, 1991; Perutz, 1970; Schulze, 1990; Wilfley et al., 1994). It is apparent, therefore, that individuals seek to be slim and fit not only to be healthy, but to be perceived by themselves and others as having desirable personal qualities (Brownell, 1991).

Women often judge all or parts of their body as if they were not right, or require rectification. They often attempt to hide or disguise parts or the whole, feel ashamed or lack confidence (Sanford, 1984). As early as the 1970s, Perutz (1970, p. 167) was reporting on fatness being a "national obsession":

> Fat is despised. Instead of signifying affluence (as it still does in poor countries), it is merely a product of it, and now indicates 'lack of self-respect.'

According to Brownell (1991) and Sams and Keels (2013), ideal body shapes in society arise from the collective influence of the mass media such as television or the internet, catalogues, clothes, advertisements, and even toys (such as Barbie). Women wishing to lose weight often have visualisations of an aesthetic ideal they'd like to attain. However:

> For many people, the ideal generates a search for an elusive goal, which often leads to poor long-term results (Wilfley et al., 1994, p. 46).

Contrary to the association of qualities such as happiness, popularity, sexiness, success and glamour with the attainment of the ideal body shape, studies have generally not supported these notions. Personal success and positive relationships are not more prevalent among thin people compared with medium-sized to overweight people (Brownell, 1991; Barsky, 1988; Glassner, 1988). Unfortunately, people perceive and judge overweight people harshly. For the individual who perceives herself, even incorrectly via body dysmorphia, to be overweight, the consequences can include body dissatisfaction, a desire to change personal body shape, lack of confidence, or eating and psychological disturbances (Coovert, Thompson, & Kinder, 1988; Smith, 1995; Noles, Cash, & Winstead, 1985; Thompson, 1990). The next section examines the aesthetically ideal body that women most often search for.

POPULAR SHAPES AND IDEALS

The desirable body image for women has become more slender over the last half century (Biddulph et al., 1984, p. 33; Hogan, 1995). Fat or overweight is definitely 'out' (van Gyn et al., 1989, p. 67). Women are at least 10 kilograms lighter than their counterparts in earlier centuries (Hogan, 1995; Niven & Carroll, 1993; Saltman, 1991). Current ideal bodies have 10–15 per cent or even less body fat, compared with 20–28 per cent for healthy women in the community (Wilfley et al., 1994, p. 45). Wilfley et al. (1994, p. 45) speculate that many of "our 'ideals' have eating disorders."

This results in a collision between cultural pressures and biological realities. According to Brownell (1991), many of the people who seek the perfect body will not attain it, or may attain it, and then lose ground.

Cultural standards for beauty and attractiveness have a major impact on women and how they perceive their bodies (Imm & Pruitt, 1991). Women are consistently judged by their physical appearance (Chernin, 1993; Saltman, 1991; Wolf, 1994). Many women are dissatisfied with their body shape and are preoccupied with having fat on their bodies. The discourse of the body involves an ideal of a thin, youthful shape, one that does not look like it has recently given birth to children (Chernin, 1981). Having a slender body is generally considered the most central and significant determinant of female attractiveness.

Centuries ago, women possessed curvaceous, rounded bodies with such ample bosoms, stomach, thighs, and bottom that they would be considered today to be overweight or unattractively fat (Cooke, 1994; Hogan, 1995; Saltman, 1991). The female figure-type expressed as most desired by men is often larger than that desired by women (Cohn et al., 1987; Paxton et al., 1991; Tiggemann & Pennington, 1990). The pressure that women feel to be slim may partly stem from the fact that women ironically believe that men prefer incredibly thin figures in women.

Dissatisfaction with one's own body shape results from the incongruence of the perceived size and shape of various body parts with that which is culturally endorsed as the ideal (van Gyn et al., 1989). According to Featherstone (1982), advertising is one source of power which has helped to create a world in which individuals are made to become emotionally vulnerable, and persuaded to adopt a critical attitude towards body, self and lifestyle. The media, including fashion advertisements, often informs women of standards that they are expected to reach in order to be acceptable (Cooke, 1994; Davis, 1985; Travis, 1988; Treble et al., 1990; Williamson, 1981). Women often feel dissatisfied and hold negative attitudes towards their bodies because they feel that their own bodies deviate too greatly from the norm (Smith, 1995).

Unfortunately, this can decrease women's degree of self-confidence, while creating more body-conscious individuals and women wishing to attain 'the look' or, at worst, perfection (Featherstone, 1982). Advertising focuses on portraying images of perfect body parts to sell different products, treating the female body as an object rather than as a whole person. If a woman is not happy with certain aspects of her figure (body), then an adverse reaction will take place and she will develop a negative feeling towards herself. This has implications for advertising and program goals in the fitness industry in general, where it is important to have women feeling good about themselves as persons. Thus, advertisements directed towards the benefits to women's well-being that is, health, fitness, and reduced stress rather than to creating 'ideal' body shapes should trigger a positive response and have greater emotional appeal.

The current prevalence of dieting, sales of diet books and enrolment of women in weight loss centres reflects the current emphasis on the slim ideal, and the idea that there is something wrong if women deviate from the stereotype modelled in magazine and television images (Chernin, 1993; Pearce, 1993; Smith, 1995). Exercise is generally viewed as an important and healthy aspect of normal weight maintenance. In moderation, it generally has a positive effect on women's body image (Berger, 1984c). Regrettably, exercise behaviours can become compulsive when they are used in pursuit of the thin stereotype.

> Vigorous exercise can be a means of weight loss or one of several tactics used by the individual to counteract the ingestion of excess calories or deal with body image concerns (Wilfley et al., 1994, p. 47).

The next section in this chapter examines the relationship between exercise and the incentive to achieve the ideal body.

BODY IMAGE AS AN INCENTIVE TO EXERCISE

The majority of women engaging in exercise programs do this for the sake of appearance or weight control (Cash et al., 1994; Davis, 1990; Krejci et al., 1992; Markula & Pringle, 2006; Silberstein et al., 1988). The pursuit of an unrealistically slim body image may give meaning to exercise behaviour (Dworkin, 2009; Redican & Hadley, 1988), but it is an unhealthy stressor for women and an inappropriate goal for a healthy exercise program (Markula, 1995).

Exercise is a socially acceptable way for an individual to deal with strong body weight concerns (Davis, 1990), compared with more radical methods such as starving and fasting, use of diet and laxative pills, induced vomiting, or submitting to cosmetic surgery (Cooke, 1994; Paxton et al., 1991). Accordingly, many women who declare inner health factors as the reason for attending the gym or even over-exercising may be attempting to provide a legitimate cover for their real commitment to altering their outer appearance (Redican & Hadley, 1988). Krejci et al. (1992) concluded that weight management does play an important role in sustained exercise behaviour in young females. For this group, missing gymnasium or fitness class sessions may be a stressor, and according to Orbach (1985), they are likely to suffer from the same sort of guilt as if they had feasted on chocolates. Women obsessed with making a body part smaller or tighter are often under an onus to attend, or a duty to conform, in order to achieve the ideal image (Redican & Hadley, 1988). However, what all women need to realise is that they are pursuing a fallacy.

Two myths surround the ideal, slim, fit body image. The first is that the body is plastic, or "infinitely malleable" (Brownell, 1991, p. 2); that it can be shaped at will towards a desired ideal. This is a myth because an individual's genes dictate that it cannot be endlessly molded to attain an "ideal" shape extensively different to the body type of the individual. The second myth is that symbolic rewards await someone who somehow achieves the body beautiful. Instant social and career success do not await!

SOCIOLOGY OF THE BODY

Foucault (1977) stated that the body is a site for the operations of power, a locus of domination through which docility is accomplished and subjectivity constituted. Discipline is a form of power that is able to transform and improve the body (Foucault, 1977). Women exercising in an attempt to control or sculpt the body are involved in a process of disciplinary techniques, and caught in the media/fitness/beauty/culture web which tells them that they must look a certain way in order to be happy and successful (Dworkin, 2009). The body is a site where the regimes of discourse and power inscribe themselves.

> Power is exercised over people through their minds, bodies and souls. The mind is a surface for the inscription of power and people submit their bodies to action and truths (Foucault, 1977, p. 102).

Women who view their bodies as falling short of the societal ideal often feel defective and decide that they must submit to dietary and exercise regimes in the quest for normalisation (Howson, 2004), or as Markula and Pringle (2006, p. 164) describe it, "aesthetic self-stylization." This is one example of the discursive control of women's bodies, subjecting women to the social norms of femininity within patriarchal boundaries.

The three categories of contemporary disciplinary practice which aim to reproduce normative femininity are:

1. Weight control to attain taut, slim bodies. Aims to produce a body of a certain size and configuration. Massiveness, power, and abundance are met with distaste. The gendering of exercise occurs, with more women than men exercising for weight control.

2. Repertoire of gestures, postures, and movements. Women must exhibit grace and poise in order to be feminine; a certain eroticism restrained by modesty (Bartky, 1988).

3. Ornamentation. This includes make-up, clothes, groomed hair, and skin care, any jewellery or body tattoos and ornamentation; all in line with current fashions and gender expectations.

These techniques secure a feminine identity "especially resistant to feminist deconstruction and revision" (Theberge, 1991, p. 128).

There has been little challenge to the two beauty myths mentioned in the previous section surrounding the ideal body for women in society. Attempts have been made by Orbach (1979), Wolf (1994), and by Cooke (1994) in Australia, to produce literature helping women to confront these myths and resist self-imposed disciplines of femininity. While women may be caught up in modes of self-observation and networks of power, never do we have to be rendered completely passive and compliant (Grosz, 1994).

However, the powerful textual discourse of femininity incorporated in women's magazines, television and advertisements presents the female body as an object of male desire and attention (Sams & Keels, 2013; Smith, 1988). The norm and cultural ideal for women is for slimness and beauty (Howson, 2004). Women are encouraged to deconstruct their bodies into parts to be improved (Duquin, 1989; Kagan & Morse, 1988; Saunders, 1994). Feeling a constant sense of lack, women search out clothing, diets, make-up, exercise, and even cosmetic surgery to bring the body into closer alignment with the textual image (Sams & Keels, 2013). In the Dove (2016) global study, the media was generally blamed for driving appearance anxiety:

> Women (69 per cent) and girls (65 per cent) cite increasing pressures from advertising and media to reach an unrealistic standard of beauty as a key force in driving appearance anxiety, while 56 per cent of all women recognize the impact of an 'always on' social media culture in driving the pressure for perfection.

Exercise class participation can help to break down notions of normative femininity as they are in opposition to traditional forms of feminine weakness. They also assist mothers to care for their own bodies and to feel greater strength and body control, as well as preventing obesity and inactivity. Classes can be designed to allow a range of fitness levels to take part, targeting enjoyment, the process of exercising, feeling healthier and improving muscle condition and function of the whole body. Women may also be part of a culture which welcomes people and allows a variety of body shapes and fitness levels to take part.

Fitness equates with being able to carry out daily activities without undue stress or fatigue. However, current advertising and media pressure has helped to alter many women's perceptions towards attainment of a beauty ideal. Qualitative research reveals that girls and women often associate fitness and exercise with slimness and sexiness (Maguire, 2008). A typical response in the study conducted by Shaw and Kemeny (1989, p. 683) was:

> Skinny = Fit so that girls can be attractive for men. Society says that women should have perfect bodies, no fat. Fitness means getting slim. Women want to lose, lose, lose.

CONCLUSION

For every woman, it may be possible to optimise individual body shape through balanced living, with healthy nutrition and exercise. This is not the equivalent of burning out through slavishly following the cult of thinness (Chernin, 1981). While morbid obesity is associated with a range of health, curves on a woman's body are natural and genetically determined (Brownell, 1991). Participation in physical activity can raise women's self-esteem, and improve body image and mental well-being (Dinucci, Finkenberg, McCune, McCune, & Mayo 1994; Kenen, 1987; Warrick & Tinning, 1989); however, it is not a passport to instant or radical body improvement. Being fit will help to moderate body fat levels, but will not achieve unrealistic goals. The natural body is not infinitely plastic; it cannot be radically reshaped. This is where some women have succumbed to plastic surgery techniques in the search for instant results (Sams & Keels, 2013).

Therefore, personal concern with body image or weight perception may motivate some women to utilise exercise as a tool in their quest for bodily perfection, rather than experiencing the pleasure of the exercise process per se, and enjoying the improvements in muscle tone, aerobic fitness, flexibility, and co-ordination of the body that may result. There is a lack of exercise programs available for women designed specifically to raise self-esteem, enhance body acceptance and to find pleasure in making the most of what they have their own bodies.

Yet while society is promoting the ideal of the body beautiful, keeping fit and staying young, working mothers have difficulty finding enough basic leisure time for themselves, let alone being able to afford the time or cost involved in extensive activities focused on self-beautification. Increasing pressures of home, family and work are reducing women's leisure time. In order for mothers to be able to participate in exercise programs, delegation of chores will have to take place to create space for such activities. To achieve this situation, women need to resist and negotiate within the interpersonal power relationships of their everyday lives, as well as in the male/female power relationships of the wider society (Wearing & Wearing, 1990).

The next chapter illustrates in greater depth the areas of power, control, and freedom in the working mother's life. To experience true leisure, women must have access to the space and freedom necessary for gaining "time out." However, certain barriers and constraints do exist in their lives which impinge on these rights. Very few authors examining the reduction of stress through exercise interventions have also appraised gender power relationships in relationship to women's participation. Chapter 5 outlines the radical nature of mothers' participation in exercise classes and reviews the work of Foucault as it relates to the issue of health and leisure for women.

Power and Disciplinary Technologies

INTRODUCTION

Women's traditional involvement in unpaid domestic labour within the household and their primary responsibility for childcare can be related to the rise of capitalism. Having women undertake a domestic role while men went out to work represented an "efficient response to the needs of production" (Dawson, 1988, p. 399). The concept of the enclosure of the individual (mother) in space (home and family) is an example underpinned by Foucault's theory of disciplinary technology (Rabinow, 1984).

Just as women's role in the productive enterprise was primarily restricted to household duties and childrearing, women's leisure was predominantly located in and oriented to home and family (Deem, 1982). The discourse of "normalised" motherhood created the reality that the roles of mother, wife and homemaker spilt over into the free time, so at any time a woman could feel:

> hurried, pressed, and strained throughout the day as a result of being perpetually 'on-call' for their husbands and children (Dawson, 1988, p. 400).

This is because the normative standard of a good mother involves a socially constructed role of someone who devotes her personal time, energy and resources to attending to the needs and welfare of her children and family:

> Central to the ideology of motherhood, then, is the notion of self-denial. For women, having children brings the expectation that they will give up or restrict their own outside involvements (e.g. job, social life, recreations, friendships) for the sake of family needs (Wimbush, 1988, p. 23).

This chapter discusses the theoretical underpinnings of this book. I outline how Foucault's theory of power and his proposed disciplinary technologies help to explain the discourse of motherhood. Women submitting themselves to an overwhelming daily schedule of tasks in an attempt to be a good mother often feel stressed from the overload and restriction. This applies both to the situation of employed mothers and mothers working at home. Foucault's theory of individual and societal observations, norms and judgements also serves to explain the creation of the discourse of ideal motherhood. Wearing's (1984) definition illustrates this concept:

Good motherhood is an ideal, assumed to be attainable only where the mother of young children withdraws from paid labour and unselfishly devotes herself to the nurture and care of her family (Wearing, 1984 in Wearing, 1989, p. 118).

While Foucault's theory of disciplinary technologies is useful, unfortunately he did not write from the woman's perspective. His gender blindness is evident in the way he treats the male experience as universal in his writing in the name of so-called gender neutrality. Nonetheless, the notion of power relations as explained by Foucault (1977) shows how women's unselfish devotion to being an ideal mother, her submission to the tasks and needs of other family members produces a docile body that may be "subjected, used, transformed, and improved" (Foucault, 1977, p. 198). The range of disciplinary technologies in play are discussed in the following section, in the context of Foucault's (1977) notion of power, as related to the lifestyles, leisure and health of working mothers.

POWER

Power is designated by a total structure of actions which incite, induce, and restrain or benefit others (Foucault, 1982b):

> In the extreme it constrains or forbids absolutely; it is nevertheless always a way of acting upon an acting subject or acting subjects by virtue of their acting or being capable of acting (Foucault, 1982b, p. 220).

Hence it "acts upon actions" (Foucault, 1982b, p. 219) or guides our conduct. Power acts over the human body and whole social field according to communication systems, habits, techniques, rules, modes of conduct and interpersonal relationships.

According to Foucault (1979b, p. 59), power acts through the family, sexual relations, and neighbourhoods. As power is intermingled with these relationships, it plays a conditioning role (Foucault, 1979a, p. 55). Its effects are explained in terms of dispositions, manoeuvres, tactics, techniques, and functions. Foucault (1977) sees power not as centrally located in the sovereign nor as an instrument of repression, but rather as a strategy that exists only when exercised. It is not necessarily operational from a top-down approach such as a dominant class and dominated class. Power is diffused throughout society at all levels (Lemert & Gillan, 1982) through a network of social relations that are constantly in tension and subject to battle. Whereas in history the sovereign power ruled supreme and discipline would often take place in the form of torture, the method used by power today is more likely to resemble that of a "panoptic gaze." Power can now take hold of bodies through operating via the conscience and sense of morality. Power exists where the body's movements are trained to become obedient, precise and efficient as exhibited in army drills or routines. This produces a "docile" body (Foucault, 1977). Power has the ability to interfere with our actions in that it can intensify the efficiency and productivity of the body (Lemert & Gillan, 1982).

The basic goal of disciplinary power was to produce a human being who could be treated as a docile body. Indeed, the Industrial Revolution and rise of capitalist society required "docile bodies" in great numbers. Disciplinary technologies or technologies of power were the preconditions for capitalism's success and they aimed to forge a "docile body that may be subjected, used, transformed and improved" (Foucault, 1977, p. 136). Foucault named the new regime of power taking hold from the eighteenth century as "bio-power" (Rabinow, 1984). According to Rabinow (1984, p. 17):

> The other pole of bio-power is the human body: the body approached not directly in its biological dimension, but as an object to be manipulated and controlled. A new set of operations, of procedures those joining of knowledge and power that Foucault calls 'technologies' come together around the objectification of the body. They form the 'disciplinary technology' that Foucault analyses in detail in *Discipline and Punish*.

The various interventions that developed for example, the growth of scientific knowledges determining what is expertly considered to be normal versus abnormal and the permeation of these ideas to produce discourses and the building up of disciplines, gave rise to the Human Sciences. The technology of power used in prisons and asylums spread to all of society. The Human Sciences are both an effect of and an instrument of this power to normalise. The disciplinary practices as found in the monasteries, houses of internment, military schools, educational institutions, prisons, hospitals, etc., were recognised by Foucault as useful techniques for the control of the population.

The technologies of power involved simple instruments to produce the required outcomes, namely "hierarchical observation," "normalised judgement," and the "examination." The chief function of the technologies was to "train" individuals that is, to transform confused, useless multitudes of bodies and forces into a multiplicity of individual and useful elements (Foucault, 1977). These instruments as referred to generally in Foucault's writing are now explained in brief.

Hierarchical Observation

Hierarchical observation involved the spatial nesting of hierarchised surveillance, and the principle employed was one of "embedding," allowing for the internal, articulated, and detailed control of the observation of individuals (Foucault, 1977, pp. 171–72):

> The goal is to make surveillance an integral part of production and control. The act of looking over and being looked over will be a central means by which individuals are linked together in a disciplinary space. The first model of this control through surveillance, efficiency through the gaze, order through spatial structure, was the military camp (Dreyfus & Rabinow, 1982, pp. 156–57).

The "spatial nesting of hierarchized surveillance" (Foucault, 1977, p. 171) is that technique used in military camps whereby housing, paths and facilities, the placement of tents and camps or even lines of soldiers, is organised in a special, defined manner such as according to rank or division. Embedding made possible the availability of detailed records, as illustrated by the records and files in hospitals of all their past and current patients. The articulated and organised system of patient surveillance makes possible the identification and classification of every patient in all of the wards, beds, floors and operating theatres. The identification tag on each patient is indeed a close level of surveillance. Schools have also employed petty mechanisms of surveillance such as having windows on the corridor side of classrooms, having half-sized toilet doors, playground supervision, roll calls, and other checking and monitoring processes (Foucault, 1977). In the workplace, supervisors and managers monitor productivity rates, Bundy clocks, absenteeism, and safety, inform directors of progress, and check for theft (Foucault, 1977).

Any training requires observation and supervision, and as this technology became more meticulous and geo-metrically dissected (including through space and time), observation moved into the subconscious. Hierarchical observations are able to function through a network of relations from top to bottom, bottom to top, and even laterally. They are discreet in that they work silently, helping to maintain standards, and have power over the body physically (Foucault, 1977). Foucault (1977) traces this process from the external physical control of torture, restraint or slavery, through to modern forms of surveillance, for instance cameras used in prisons, locked doors in asylums, and self-restraints in terms of sexuality, eating habits and moral laws. For according to Foucault (1977, p. 30), "The soul is the effect and instrument of a political anatomy; the soul is the prison of the body." Strict self-discipline and surveilling oneself for appropriate behaviours became a virtue for example, a housewife comparing the meal she has prepared with the recipe pictures in a "women's magazine," or a woman her own body shape with that of a model appearing on television.

Normalising Judgement

New technologies of power appearing in society aimed to control the body and soul of individuals. Therefore:

> Through the specification of the most detailed aspects of everyday behaviour, almost anything could be potentially punishable. The nonconformist, even the temporary one, became the object of disciplinary attention (Dreyfus & Rabinow, 1982, p. 158).

Even trivial areas of life were now captured by power and deviations to the expected norm subject to micro-penalties of time, activity, behaviour, speech, body, and sexuality (Foucault, 1977). Originally, micro-penalties were enforced in the workshop, school and army, for example for the following discrepancies or deviancies:
- time

- lateness
- absences
- interruptions or delays to task completion

- activity

  - inattention

  - negligence

  - lack of zeal

- behaviour

  - impoliteness

  - disobedience

- speech

  - idle chatter

  - insolence

- body

  - 'incorrect' attitudes

  - irregular gestures

  - lack of cleanliness

- sexuality

  - impurity

  - indecency (Foucault, 1977, p. 178).

The slightest deviation from what was considered correct behaviour subjected one to punishment. Procedures of punishment included light physical punishment to minor deprivations and petty humiliations. If one did not reach the expected norms or behaviours at one's predetermined standard or developmental level for example, by failing an exam then one was punished for nor fulfilling one's "potential." Therefore "normalising judgement" subordinated people and induced docility through ensuring that attention was given by people to their work, study, and self-discipline. Strategies utilised by this technology of power include:

- grading, marking, setting norms;

- providing a hierarchy of qualities, skills and aptitudes (so evident in today's push for the setting of occupational/job 'competency-based standards');

- judging excellence versus mediocrity versus failure;

- comparing and differentiating;

- conforming, grouping, grading and pressuring to conform (Foucault, 1977, p. 181).

It is interesting that the large-scale study on mothers' health carried out by a global pharmaceutical company acknowledged the high levels of stress commonly experienced. However, ironically on the same website, vitamins are advertised to this same group of women, with the statement, "we understand you do not always put yourself first" (Cenovis, 2017).

The Examination

The examination maintained the control of individuals and the subjection of power:

> It is a normalizing gaze, a surveillance that makes it possible to qualify, to classify, and to punish. It establishes over individuals a visibility through which one differentiates them and judges them (Foucault, 1977 in Rabinow, 1984, p. 197).

It increased visibility of individuals and reinforced the power exercised over them: "It is this fact of surveillance, constant visibility, which is the key to disciplinary technology" (Dreyfus & Rabinow, 1982, p. 159). The examination was a "mechanism of power relations making possible the extraction and constitution of knowledge" (Foucault, 1977, p. 185), and "surrounded by all its documentary techniques, it makes each individual a case" (Foucault, 1977, p. 191).

Through this building up of dossiers about individuals, and the increased scientification of knowledge came the birth of the Clinical Sciences. Power had produced knowledge and truth, as explained by Foucault (1988, p. 106):

> What struck me, in observing the human sciences, was that the development of all these branches of knowledge can in no way be dissociated from the exercise of power generally speaking, the fact that societies can become the object of scientific observation, that human behaviour became, from a certain

point on, a problem to be analyzed and resolved, all that is bound up, I believe, with mechanisms of power. So, the birth of the human sciences goes hand in hand with the installation of new mechanisms of power.

All of these techniques of power are present at every level of society and utilised by very diverse institutions (for example, the family, the army, schools, police) and between individuals (Foucault, 1980a in Rabinow). Further, the processes of hierarchized observation and normalised judgement serve to create the discourse of ideal motherhood, whereby women submit themselves to internalised self-examination and surveillance. The effect on one's leisure of being a full-time housewife was very negative; the fact that so many women were at home added to the psychological pressure that housewives ought to be doing the housework, not taking time out to play. However, power relationships are neither static nor one-way and, by inference, there is some room to move for women, some relative autonomy in each situation (Wearing, 1990).

RESISTANCE

Power runs through the social network and acts to bring about effects. Power is in play in all areas of our life and it risks losing or winning ground, just like share values on the stock exchange: "Power is won like a battle and lost in just the same way" (Foucault, 1979b, p. 60). Power is "never totally on one side or from one point of view," and at every moment "power is in play in small individual parts" (Foucault, 1979b, p. 60). This notion of power implies a better chance for transformation than does opposition to an all-dominating force. Another major characteristic of power that Foucault proposed is that freedom must exist for power to be exerted (Foucault, 1982b, p. 221), "Since without the possibility of recalcitrance, power would be equivalent to a physical determination," or that of a person held in chains: "Power is exercised over free subjects and only insofar as they are free" (Foucault, 1982b, p. 221).

Therefore, there are no relations of power without the possibility of resistances. Resistance, like power, exists in multiple and global strategies (Foucault, 1979a). Hence, where power exercises itself in a network field of force relations—even through means of class, race, religion, gender and age—resistance is possible. One is never trapped in every way by power and points of resistance are present everywhere (Foucault, 1979a). This can occur through effective regroupings or recalcitrance, especially at vulnerable points, to the dominant discourse (Weedon, 1987).

The most powerful discourses have firm, institutional bases, as illustrated by law, social welfare, education and work. Yet these can also be sites for contest or challenge (Weedon, 1987). For example, equal employment opportunity, affirmative action, pushes for equal pay between men and women and the introduction of paid maternity leave or more flexible work arrangements for women and mothers illustrate changes possible through resistance, challenge, negotiation and arbitration. As discourses can be sites for contradiction, they provide the discursive means to resist (Weedon, 1987). Initial struggles for change or redefinitions of what we commonly accept as the norm can take place in the consciousness of the individual (Weedon, 1987).

The discourse of motherhood includes acceptable roles, standards, and an ethic of care (Weedon, 1987). Leisure is one aspect of life where mothers can resist ideal definitions of "mother," "carer," or "wife" (Wearing & Wearing, 1990, p. 163). However, in order to create space for such leisure activities, women may have to negotiate or resist in their interpersonal and other social relations. Ultimately, it is the individual who either acts or does not act.

Leisure as Resistance

The prospect of mothers engaging in leisure purely for pleasure is antithetical to societal expectations that we should put others' needs before our own (Lenskyj, 1991). This is illustrated in the situation where women with paid work involvement in addition to home duties such as childcare and domestic roles may feel guilty and not entitled to access leisure time before having first completed all chores or tended to the needs of children (Lenskyj, 1991).

In a patriarchal society, women often end up combining work with their leisure for example, ironing while watching television, or caring for children and entertaining them with games while gardening (Lenskyj, 1991).

> While unpaid labour is equated with leisure and while motherhood is equated with selfless devotion to the needs of others, leisure in the sense of 'freely chosen, self-enhancing activity' or of 'my space' is obtained only with difficulty (Wearing, 1989, p. 118).

The negative effects of these overwhelming, constant demands on women, which leave them with no time to think or to express their own individuality or to have "time out," are problematic to women's mental health (Wimbush, 1986). Henderson et al. (1989, p. 78) proposed that:

> Through leisure, in which the essence of the experience is one of choice, women can learn to value themselves as individuals and challenge some of the societal restrictions and stereotypes. Leisure participation for women, therefore, could be a means of liberation from restrictive gender roles and social scripts, and thus, a means of empowerment.

Power, according to Foucault, forms knowledge and produces discourse. Resistance can involve the uprising of knowledges previously discredited. Feminism seeks to discover and change the subtle and deep-seated causes of women's oppression (Carpenter & Sheklow, 1985). The establishment of leisure as a valid concept for women, and the notion of leisure as an outlet for mothers to deservedly experience and feel the freedom associated with leisure, are examples of subjugated judgements that have the potential to form alternative and yet legitimate discourses for women.

> The essence of the power relationship is not to discover what we are, but to refuse what we are and to reach toward what we could be, claims Foucault (Wearing, 1990, p. 41).

Leisure is an opportunity for women to resist the "normalising" gaze of stereotyped motherhood ideologies. It also implies control and a greater sense of space for women. Space is fundamental to resistance. Foucault suggests the need for "heterotopias," those singular spaces to be found in some given social spaces whose functions are different or even the opposite of others (Foucault, 1982a in Rabinow, 1984, p. 252). Even when feminist discourses lack the social power to realise their versions of knowledge in institutional practices, "They can offer a discursive space from which the individual can resist dominant subject positions" (Weedon, 1987, p. 110).

We might not be able to transform workplaces overnight into spaces that offer crèches and exercise classes at lunchtimes. Hope for gradual improvement in leisure opportunities may rest with each woman negotiating for these developments at work. At the micro level, mothers can delegate household or childcare tasks to a partner, opt for take-away or have a teen cook the meal. This can create a sense of time off from the motherhood role. Personal changes devised by 100 women I interviewed in focus group research, intended as strategies to be immediately incorporated into their lifestyles as a means to help reduce stress, included:

1. taking time out and 'giving' to self-more

2. delegating tasks

3. not feeling guilty (about paid work involvement or the 'state' of the housework)

4. reassessing roles, not aiming to be a 'super-mum'/enjoying 'quality' time with spouse or partner

5. relaxing/being more positive

6. communicating more/being sensitive to others (e.g. not criticising husband's effort or results when helping with a household task)

7. obtaining household help

8. exercising more

9. time management (Pearce, 1989, p. 14).

Leisure experiences can be "self-enabling, raising the self-esteem of women and give individual women some power" (Wearing & Wearing, 1988, p. 121). Once women experience the benefits of leisure and understand that it is their right to regularly access it, they may then realise that it is one sphere where space for themselves can be created and male power is held at bay (Wearing & Wearing, 1988). Resistance at the individual level is the first step in the production of alternative forms of knowledge or discursive spaces, and gradually increasing social power.

The right of mothers to their own leisure space and 'time out' from domestic and/or outside home duties will hopefully evolve to a legitimate entitlement and normal discourse in the eyes of society. This can only occur if there is a shift in gender/power relationships. Feminists have been considering the transformance of how we see power and the body. Previously, feminists have sought equality on grounds of the mind, and now some researchers see the retrieval of the female body as a source of power. The body is not passive; it can be a source of resistance and power constructed by discourse (Grosz, 1991).

The body may be seen as active, not passive. It is a social surface of political inscriptions as we live through and are constructed by discourses. The body may no longer be seen as a-cultural as it makes a difference to how we "wear" and act out our gender identity and roles. This is a transformance from a mind/body split (Grosz, 1991). Many feminists now understand the benefits of this transformation, as previous bi-polar analyses often placed the mind in opposition with the body. Rescuing females from biological definitions and giving them access to a definition based on their lived experiences, activities and roles will do more to account for the specific disciplinary practices that women are subjected to (Grosz, 1994). It also implies that the mind cannot be made useful without the body, and that the body is a site for inscriptions of power and resistance a concept utilised to help explain the women's experiences reported in this book.

Three main areas where Foucault and feminism converge are:

1. Both identify the body as a site of power. The body can be a locus of domination through which docility is accomplished and subjectivity constituted. The body is also capable of resistance or opposition.

2. Both point to local and intimate operations of power ('the personal is political'), rather than focusing exclusively on the supreme power of the state.

3. Feminism and Foucault identify the role of discourse in sustaining power, and the challenges contained within marginalised or un-recognised discourses (Diamond & Quinby, 1988, p. x).

If women can engage in more positive leisure experiences, they may feel greater empowerment, autonomy, and self-esteem. Leisure offers an outlet for women to challenge some aspects of their subordination. The renegotiation and resistance by women as they take time out and make space for themselves to do as they please involve the insurrection of subjugated knowledges, a challenge to the dominant discourse of motherhood, and the re-examination of what is considered "normal."

When mothers resist to make their own space for leisure or for their own socialising, they can perceive that taking this regular leisure time does not take away from them being a "good" mother. This is illustrated in Figure 5.1. To reach this stage, mothers need to give themselves permission and reassurance that "it's OK," as explained by this dual-career mother:

One of the reasons that I have so much difficulty making time for myself, doing things I want to do even if I consider them frivolous, has to do with not being able to give myself the most basic thing - approval (Shank, 1986, p. 313).

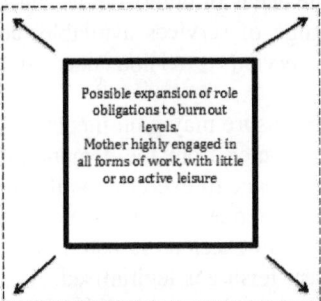

Situation A: Lifestyle of working mother – limiting in forms of constraints for leisure opportunities or to take time-out. Women obligated through ethic of care and self-discipline to be family-centred. Role overload can occur with increasing responsibilities and stress levels.

Possible expansion of role obligations to burn out levels.
Mother highly engaged in all forms of work with little or no active leisure

Situation B: Leisure as resistance leads to easing of stress levels and feelings of greater wellbeing

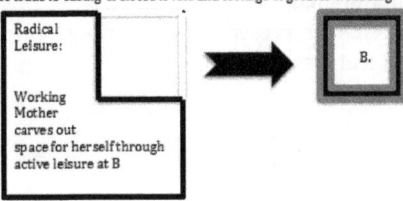

Radical Leisure:

Working Mother carves out space for herself through active leisure at B

B.

Situation C. Re-negotiation of tasks has occurred, along with government–sponsored leisure and childcare facilities, enabling mothers to have greater access to leisure

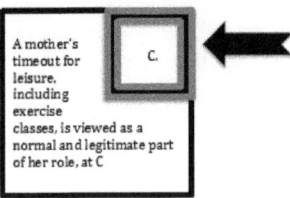

A mother's time out for leisure, including exercise classes, is viewed as a normal and legitimate part of her role, at C

C.

Figure 5.1: Leisure as Resistance.

Through mothers just giving themselves this basic approval, perhaps more women could engage in leisure. Leisure can be a source of self-nurturance, recuperation and renewal if the desire for this space or time out is materialised via strategies of negotiation, resistance or recognition of self-worth. Strategies of resistance might include delegating chores to husband or children; learning to ask for help; having days off to rest; naps; learning to say no; learning that leisure time is a personal right; letting children be more responsible for themselves; creating buddy systems whereby women take leisure together and help out with childcare; shutting the bathroom door and enjoying a long relaxing bath; opting for take-away or having the family prepare meals.

CONCLUSION

Gender role expectations and socialisation can interfere with the process of taking time out for leisure or the willingness to reward one's self in this manner. Strong conflictual feelings can interfere with nurturing one's self due to the ethic of care and emphasis on attending to the needs of others before our own. Structural changes, such as improvements in the range of services available, accessibility, childcare, safety, and training of staff in service provision may also enhance women's leisure involvement.

Mothers who engage in leisure may gain mental well-being and easing of stress. The periodic need to find distance from the demanding roles of mother and worker can be satisfied by finding a space to exercise, as illustrated by Figure 5.1. The need for changes in socialisation practices, whereby mothers who give to themselves by taking time out to exercise are not seen as selfish, is very important. This is illustrated at point C in Figure 5.1 where leisure is legitimised. As a society, we must continue to reinforce the idea that it is acceptable and healthy for working mothers to receive as well as give nurturance.

The next chapter presents stories from real mothers about how exercise helps them cope and feel less stressed.

CHAPTER 6

Exercise for Stress Relief: Subjective Experiences of Mothers

ACCORDING TO MOTHERS, DOES EXERCISE HELP THEM COPE WITH STRESS?

In this chapter, I include compelling accounts given by mothers as to how they believe participating in exercise classes helps them to effectively cope with stress. For the group of mothers, I surveyed for this book, exercise was noted by all but two of the participants as helping them to relax and manage their stated levels of stress.

When invited to describe whether exercise helps them cope with stress, typical responses from the participating mothers most commonly indicated a type of relaxation response:

- Exercise lets out the stress and helps me to relax.

- It makes me feel relaxed and happy that I've actually exercised.

- Yes, (exercise) helps me relax, takes my mind off other problems.

- Takes my mind off worries. Releases pent up frustrations.

- Lowers my stress feelings. Helps me cope better. Helps me relax.

- Yes, it helps, as I totally forget all my worries when I come to this class. It enables you to release stored up frustrations vent your anger.

- Definitely yes. I feel a lot calmer after the class.

- Gives me a break, puts my mind on other things. The class alleviates these feelings of stress as I feel better able to cope mentally and physically.

- Improves my general well-being as the work out releases tension and makes you feel good. Calms me down and helps me focus on other things.

- Makes me feel good. Definitely relieves stress.

- Exercise helps me cope with stress for a short while.

- Calm and relaxed and able to cope with the rest of the day.

- Feel good, feel a sense of achievement that I've actually done something.

- Very healthy and feeling good within myself after doing exercises.

- Relaxed clear mind.

- After the class, I felt like I could keep coping.

- You do not get as stressed as easily.

For all but two of the women, the class left them feeling invigorated, with more energy, purpose, and strength to cope than before. For example, when I met Vera, she was quite specific in explaining to me that she feels much healthier and is coping with life in general more effectively after taking part in exercise classes:

> Certainly, for me, it helped me mostly have a look at myself, and how I needed to make sure I managed my stress, and exercise was good for that. After the class, I felt I could go on and do more or just go and do something different. I can rush for a bus or to a shop and I'm not puffing and panting like I used to. And mentally I feel clearer.

Sue also highlighted the difference in how she felt after the class compared with beforehand:

> Before I was pretty hassled, trying to get there and getting the kids to school and everything, but afterwards, I'd just feel healthier and I'd eat a healthy lunch rather than just grab something on the run. I just feel cooler in the mind and really good, more in control.

TIME OUT: EXERCISE FORMS A BREAK OR DISTRACTION FROM DAILY STRESSORS

For the mothers participating in exercise classes, taking part was described as a mechanism for relieving anxiety. From a process of positive immersion in the activity, the mothers could dissolve frustrations and distract themselves from daily stressors. It generally "lifted away" any tensions. The most common explanations given for the mechanism behind exercise helping mothers cope with stress included that it formed a "stress release" and a break away from normal stressors. Typical responses included:

- Because I am away from day to day housework.

- Takes your mind off your worries.

- Releases pent up frustrations.

- It's time away to think about myself.

- Yes, (exercise) relaxes muscles and gives me a break from everything.

- I had never thought of exercising for stress until coming to this class. I have now found a wonderful way to cope.

- It's my time and it uses up extra energy in exercise instead of anger by having a clearer mind to put thing in perspective.

A few mothers described feeling tired after the class, but this was characterised as a positive type of tiredness:

- Tired and positive. Tired but happy.

- Satisfied. A little tired.

- Relaxed, refreshed, pleasantly tired (sometimes).

- Excellent tired and I feel relaxed.

Taking part in exercise classes helps mothers to cope with stress because it helps dissolve anxieties and tension. Merron explained that after the class she did not worry about things so much:

> I feel like I've, ah, exercised my stress away, um, more relaxed, like things that were worrying me before I got there, I somehow got them out of my system. Because I exercised or whatever, they did not seem to worry me as much.

Lesley described exercise as helping her cope with stress because "it gives her a break, and puts her mind on other things." Evelyn believes that because of the exercise, she is able to cope more effectively throughout the day:

Yes, exercise helps. It calms me down and helps me focus on other things. I usually feel tense and jittery before the class from getting the children organized for school, (however) straight after the class I feel calm and relaxed, and feel able to cope with the rest of the day.

Letting go, even temporarily, of the ethic of care, including overriding concerns about any scheduled tasks, work or other worries dominating the mother's mind, was a common theme to emerge when I sought to discover how the exercise class reduced stress levels. Once the mother was participating in the class, it formed an enjoyable and effective stress-relieving distraction.

THE EXERCISE IS FOR THE MOTHERS THEMSELVES

The classes formed an activity that took place away from work, reserved just for the mother herself. For example, Karen explained that the main benefit she achieves from the classes is "freedom on her own." To further illustrate this point, Merron thought the reason she felt more relaxed after taking part in a class was due to "giving back" to herself, after giving so much of herself to others non-stop, around the clock:

Well, firstly I think it is because I am doing it for me, so I feel a lot better. Secondly, it's obviously doing me good at the same time.

This is in resistance to the ideology of motherhood which states that a mother should be available to others, or on stand-by, not away from the home doing something like this. Normally, mothers can feel pressure to put everyone else's needs first. The theme of giving back to self was illustrated by the following comments:

- The class gives time for me.

- It is time for myself and I enjoy it.

- Freedom on my own.

- Doing something for me letting it all out.

- Physical and feeling of 'doing it just for me.'

- Feels good and I know it was for me; my time.

- It's time away to think about myself. There's no other ways available to cope with stress yet, as children too young and too much going on at home.

- Feeling like I'm doing something for myself instead of staying home like a home-bound mother. I am feeling my age and feeling young, feeling my body react to exercise and feeling good about myself and my body again.

Jenny feels "pleased within herself" after the class. She explained to me that, through taking part in regular exercise classes, she felt better able to cope with minor crises and thought she was developing more patience:

> Yes, you calm right down. Like one time there was this girl, I went to this shop last week at a particular shopping Centre, and she was really rude; she's always rude. So, one time after classes I went and I was served by her and it did not worry me. I just thought, 'Poor girl, she's got a problem.' So that's how it affects me.

Sarah confided in me that through participating in the class, she could feel better, even after a particularly rough day at the office:

> I think you start to concentrate on what you're doing in the exercise class, you see other people that you do know and you start to laugh a bit and somehow it all disappears when you start to do the class.

Kathy is a 35 year-old mother of three children. She said her main reason for attending exercise classes was for personal stress. At the time of joining our group she was having counselling for a recent sexual assault. Combined with osteopathic massage and exercise classes, she believed it had helped her to cope better. When I asked Kathy if the classes help in any way to alleviate stress or anxiety, she replied:

> Very much so. One, it's my time. Two, it uses extra energy in exercise instead of towards anger, [giving me] a clearer mind to put things in perspective. [It] gets me out of bed for the day I can cope with more in one day.

Other means of achieving time out from everyday responsibilities that the exercising mothers recommended as being effective for stress relief included:

- naps

- float tanks.

- sitting in the garden.

- calligraphy class.

- 4.00pm 'Playschool Cocktail' Gin and Ice Cream.

- a bath before bedtime.

- cappuccinos with friends.

(Though one participant said, "No other way was possible," compared with exercise classes). Merron had even recommended exercise classes as a method of coping to her own neighbour up the street who had been having a difficult time at home and is "stressed out":

> I did not realise till after I went to your class, probably because of the situation I am in, how much better I felt afterwards, so I would definitely recommend it to other mums, just to see the difference it made.

CONCLUSION

Feeling a sense of time out from one's stressful lifestyle and normal role distracts mothers from stressors and allows them to assume a different role in their own space, in their own time, at their leisure. Individuals with the poorest health states commonly experience feelings of powerlessness to make choices about their own lives. However, the greatest levels of subjective well-being are experienced by those mothers feeling the greatest amount of control over their own lives (Currie, 2009).

The roles of "good wife" and "mother" exert an invasive influence over the spare time activities of women (APS, 2015). Exercise classes provide an opportunity for resistance through the capacity of a mother to reject labels and constraints and act to change her existing condition, for instance if that involves having little time to self, or lack of leisure. Through involving herself in leisure, a woman has the opportunity to take responsibility for herself and her time. Through a process of positive immersion and time out, she can rid herself, even if only temporarily, of her "working mother" role while engaging in leisure (while someone else performs childcare). Exercise classes offer mothers a temporary freedom and a mechanism to reduce feelings of tension and stress.

According to the point of view of the exercising mothers, the classes were a ready means of alleviating stress, and could be used as a strategy to negotiate a space of their own. Chapter 7 delves further into how exercise participation may be explained in terms of resistance by some participants, as a means of escape from the day-to-day grind and caring role of being a mother.

Exercise as a Source of Resistance

INTRODUCTION

Households constitute their own form of power and domination over women's work, time, leisure, and space. The regulatory controls of "bio-politics" encompass the "vast array of (repressive) collective measures undertaken to regulate the population" (Harvey & Sparks, 1991, p. 169). Households are just one social institution providing the discipline, techniques of power and sets of conditions that coerce, control and train bodies. The internalised norm or intrinsic attitude that it is the mother's responsibility to do the caring, cleaning, cooking and most other unpaid work is a disciplinary technique or principle that dictates women's roles and bodies. It creates what Foucault (1977) calls "docile bodies."

This method or technique of disciplining the body as a productive machine increases its usefulness and docility, for instance, a housewife slaving away endlessly without complaint. Control of docile bodies that is, of mothers in the home involves such techniques as:

1. The labelling or identification of private spaces; for instance, spaces in the home such as the kitchen and laundry being allocated as "women's spaces."

2. Coding's, expectations, and social mores automatically assigning or aligning certain tasks such as cleaning or cooking to women as they're viewed as a woman's domain.

3. Routinisation of daily schedules; for example, women submitting themselves to long lists of unpaid work tasks, household rituals or a specified order of tasks, and "best practice" methods utilised to complete those chores to the highest standard (Rojek, 1985).

This form of power over women is neither hierarchical (imposed from the top), nor foundational (arising from determinate social relations such as class relations). Rather, it arises in a capillary fashion from below, expressed through people's knowledge and social relations for example, their understandings, perceptions, beliefs and practices concerning gender-appropriate physical activity and roles (Harvey & Sparks, 1991).

The body is central to Foucault's analysis and is a site of constant struggle. As a mother is a thinking, feeling subject capable of resistance and innovations, she is also a subject able to reflect upon the discursive relations which constitute her and the society in which she lives and choose from the options available (Weedon, 1987, p. 125). Some critics have rejected Foucault's work because they claim his analyses offer little hope of an individual resisting, changing, or reforming a system that might be deemed oppressive (Racevskis, 1993, p. 102). However, according to Foucault, our freedom exists more in our ability to transform our relationship to traditional ways of being, rather than in being able to control the direction that the future will take. One person does not "control the overall direction of history," but is able to choose among the discourses and practices available to them and use them creatively (Sawicki, 1991, p. 103).

Power circulates in a social field of struggle on and by individuals over others as well as themselves. Freedom can lie in rebelling against those ways in which we are already defined, categorised and classified. Therefore, mothers can resist the 'normal' ideology or notion of mothering by:

- taking time out for well-deserved leisure

- "sharing the caring"

- negotiating with other family members for them to take some responsibility

- resisting overload and guilt wherever possible and realising that time to self, time to exercise or be with friends, is a well-deserved personal right.

Leisure provides the potential for empowerment and personal choice to help mothers value themselves and gain the confidence to challenge society's gender role stereotypes. When women exercise, it allows them to create a new space which provides a means for them to escape both physically and mentally from feelings of entrapment and obligation. In this chapter, using the mothers' own descriptions and words, I illustrate what this concept means to the mothers themselves. The exercise classes helped mothers to empower themselves because they used it as period of 'time out' to stop what they were doing, and to focus on something completely different.

USING EXERCISE FOR LEISURE AS SPACE AND EMPOWERMENT: THE WOMEN'S STORIES

"Resurrecting the subjugated knowledges" (Sawicki, 1991, p. 31) of women's leisure experiences and their access to leisure is crucial to women's sense of empowerment. When mothers take time out to exercise, they redefine their normal traditional role (or as much of this ideology as they willingly or unwillingly live up to) of being on call 24 hours a day. For example, Merron told me that during the class she was able to use exercise as a stress filter to forget her usual worries and "get them out of [her] system."

Penny was another mother who explained to me how she felt she could escape from her regular existence through the classes. Penny is 27 years old, with a young child. Doing something for herself was very important, and she enjoyed the good feelings she gained from exercise. When I enquired about current stressors in Penny's life, she replied:

> Really Janet, you do not want to know; but to be honest I have a brother who I do not see or hear from due to a feud. Another brother with a life-threatening disease. My husband's brother has cancer, another one with medically acquired AIDS. My grandmother has suffered a stroke and is angry and resentful, apart from other problems such as home, income, Christmas et cetera. I am suffering a lot from stress and I was getting severe headaches.

As time went by, Penny began to feel more motivated to attend the exercise classes because she could, in her words, "feel good in herself." She explained to me how she looked forward to the class beforehand, and "really enjoyed it," as she could escape from her normal or usual daily existence:

> Yes, the class does help to a degree, I can come here and forget who I really am and escape to another being, another person. The music played a big factor. If it was loud and if I liked it, it made it easy to forget problems and fantasies. I felt young again, free again, forgot everyday life.

Many mothers described the class as being a time when they could assume a role which was not that of 'working mother.' A common theme was that the class represented a time or place where the mother could be completely free, forget about troubles, and clear the mind of any anxiety or tension:

- If I have done my class or walked and I come in to do some administration, my mind's cleared. I feel much better overall and in feelings of well-being.

- Yes, it helps, as I totally forget all my worries when I come to this class.

- Yes, I feel good about myself because I am actually doing it for me and hence feel good all over. Emotionally it helps you forget about your troubles. So, I might arrive feeling perhaps angry or frustrated about something, so I decide to take it out on the class and I feel relieved for a while.

- Oh, [you] just sort of feel better in the mind, really. You're feeling like you're doing something for yourself.

The claiming of a new space, designated as being just for the mother herself, was explained by the mothers as making them feel happier and more accomplished. For example, Vera is 49 years old with 4 grown-up children and in full-time employment. She described how taking the time out from her busy job to do the exercise class was "a good idea," as her previous counselling position had left her close to "burn-out." Vera explained that she had adjusted her lifestyle, telling me she had "changed her personal philosophy," in that she did not want to put that sort of pressure on herself anymore. Residing at a local community centre which was also her workplace meant that it was difficult to differentiate between "work space" and "home space":

> Janet: What do you find is the main source of your stress?
>
> Vera: I found that it was hard, living on the premises, to disassociate from work, and so the exercises really helped me in that it helped me switch off from work.
>
> Janet: What did you think of the classes?
>
> Vera: I thought the exercises were a really good idea and they made me take a look at myself and how I needed to manage my stress; and exercise was good for that.

Attending the exercise class helped Vera break free from her work space, switch off, and escape to a space of her own. Vera believed that to achieve a distinction in her mind between the two spaces was essential. Without a separate space for herself, she could feel her stress levels "creeping" up:

> It's really critical that I take my private space, but because I like the job and I like people, et cetera, et cetera, et cetera, [laughs] I find that very gradually it was creeping up and I was letting it [the job] impose on me.

Vera explained to me how she was able to switch off from her work space, which was so close to her home space, to a totally individual space, due to her exercise involvement:

> Well, once the music starts, and I get into the exercise, I just find that I'm in a totally different, you know, [pause] space. Rather than at work, which you know is really good. And the feeling of enthusiasm that I get from you is just great.

Exercising allowed the women the chance to be in control of their minds and bodies, and not submit themselves to endless household chores or work for a change. Personal well-being could be the new priority. These elements of freedom and choice are central features of both leisure and feminism (Henderson et al., 1989). Sarah felt that the class acted as a filter that helped her to rid herself of any negative emotions, and reward herself for working so hard during the day:

Sarah: I feel that it does something good for me because when you come
          from work you relax by doing that [exercises], and um, if you have
          any frustrations from work, you get rid of them in class.

Janet: What sort of frustrations might you feel from work?

Sarah: You can be a bit tense, you can be a bit stressed, you can have some
          bad customers, angry customers that you have been upset about and
          that helps when you do exercise.

Sarah noticed that if she had a headache, it disappeared during the class:

Janet: A really bad headache?

Sarah: Yeah, a migraine type.

Janet: What, straight away?

Sarah: Well, I think once you've warmed up and then the blood starts to
          circulate really fast.

Merron told me how she enjoyed rewarding herself by attending the class after the
strain of juggling multiple roles all day long. She said it was:

Doing something for me. After running around doing everything for the kids
I actually feel like I am doing something for me, and I think getting out with
other mums and just mixing as a group.

The sense of time out was able to be achieved alone or with other friend's present.
Julie believed that in order to gain time out for herself, she did not have to do things
on her own:

I can go and do a sport with other people. It's nice to meet other ladies and
have a talk.

However, from the perspective of the mothers, time out is most effective when
childcare is available. Depending on regular attendance and effort made, it appears
that the process of attending the classes and interacting with other women, combined
with gains in strength and stamina, contributed greatly to a participant's redefinition
of her own capabilities. To illustrate, Julie told me that as a result of the benefits she
felt from attending the classes, she had redefined her self-boundaries and limitations:

Janet: What do you feel you achieve from the classes?

Julie: As I went along, just the feeling of getting fit, things I could do at the end [of the program] that I certainly could not do at the beginning, just the satisfaction. You feel like a more rounded person. I've always enjoyed taking part in life rather than sitting back and watching it go past. My life has to revolve around goals, and part of that is being fit and healthy.

THE REWARD FOR SELF IN GAINING GREATER CONTROL

Both feminism and leisure revolt against domination and encourage freedom of choice, not restrictions or limitations. The women who participated in exercise classes for leisure told me over and over again that they felt in greater control.

A common theme was that they felt rewarded for taking part by a sense of achievement and accomplishment. Gaining control of one's body and one's life is a major goal of feminism. The mothers taking part in fitness classes felt better about themselves and expressed a greater sense of confidence and individual control:

- If l keeps fit I feel good about myself.

- Makes you feel good and more confident.

- Makes me feel good.

- I feel more confident.

- I feel good just to be able to achieve just getting there. It improves my self-esteem.

- If I go regularly, yes, I am happier about my body and then in turn feel fitter, which gives me energy to 'bounce' through the day.

- I lost weight, gained self-esteem, and also felt like I achieved something each time.

All of the mothers I interviewed for this book admitted at some stage to experiencing feelings of stress caused by the constraints placed upon them by their multiple roles. When they are able to choose to participate in exercise classes, they described feeling in greater control, refreshed from their experience and less tense or anxious as a result. When asked if exercise helped them cope with stress, many agreed it most definitely did because they could identify a real sense of coping associated with feeling generally happier, healthier and better about themselves:

- Improves general well-being as the work out releases tension and makes you feel good.

- I always come away from class feeling very relaxed and pleased with myself.

- The class alleviates these feelings of stress, as I feel better able to cope mentally and physically.

- I feel fitter and healthier.

- Helped you cope with day to day matters more easily as well as having time out for yourself.

- It is for me time out. It makes me think of good things and takes my mind off the stresses.

- If I can maintain a good fitness level I am generally happier within.

- afterwards I feel great for hours and in the long term I feel I'm helping my overall feeling of well-being; must be endorphins or something.

- Yes, I feel positive after the class with a brighter outlook about things.

Amy elaborated further on feeling better after the class, saying:

> Oh, I feel heaps better because I've done my exercise and just probably got rid of a lot of frustration that's in my body. I always feel good after the class. I just think it's important for your health and mental fitness. It just helps you get through the day a lot easier and just makes you feel a lot better.

She also pointed out to me that, "Women who have not done it before might not know the difference."

Belinda is 49 years of age, with two adult children. She discussed with me how she believed that mothers have to learn to shift the boundaries of constraint in their life and take time out to exercise to feel greater control and well-being. She decided long ago to resist the notion that she was always going to be a supermom, which involved the stressful burden of living out multiple roles successfully, with no respite. Belinda talked about her active lifestyle and how exercise is an extremely important part of her life. She expressed the belief that all mothers need to take time out to exercise, do something for themselves and reap the benefits; however, she acknowledged the constraints existing for many first-time mothers with children.

Belinda enjoys the self-discipline and fitness rewards that she gains from regular exercise. She participates in aerobics, golf, power walking and walking with the dog. When I asked Belinda if there were any stressors in her life at the moment, she replied that it was only her mother, whom she has to help care for as she has Parkinson's disease. This was Belinda's only main worry, except for her daughter's occasional relationship traumas. Belinda's access to personal resources meant that even if it was raining, she could use her own home gym or exercise bike.

Belinda often stressed during our interviews the importance, in her opinion, for all mothers to access regular exercise. In her opinion, it formed part of a basic healthy lifestyle regime. She recommended it to other women as a way to help them to forget about their stress. However, she also maintained that the classes should offer childcare in order to be accessible for all.

> Janet: How important is getting that time out every day for woman's health?
>
> Belinda: Very. Extremely. At least half an hour to yourself. Relaxation and a feeling of well-being for you. Some people get a kick out of getting their hair or nails done. It's a reward. It's something for yourself. And it's for you, whereas it's not for anyone else, you know, cause you're a mother, and you're a wife, and an auntie. This is just for you.
>
> Janet: Do you think women feel it's a right for them?
>
> Belinda: Not enough. Not enough women do because they're nurturers, they're givers, and you've got to draw the line.
>
> Janet: How did you learn to do that? How did you develop that philosophy?
>
> Belinda: Maturity. When you're younger you're busy all the time. And it's not till you're older that you get to think that, 'Do I want to be healthy longer?'.

I really gained a strong impression that Belinda was definitely in touch with her own rights to personal health. However, she acknowledged that she had only been able to exercise this right since her children had become independent.

Julie was another participant who described her involvement in terms of "satisfaction, commitment, and achievement." She viewed the classes as a goal she had fulfilled and explained the satisfaction she experienced in taking part as being due to improvements in personal fitness, a break from home and family, a way to do something for herself and the boost it had given her self-esteem.

> Janet: Mentally, what do the classes do for you?
>
> Julie: As I said, I like to get in and do a lot with my life, and one, it made me feel that I was fitter, I could actually see that I had lost weight, I could see the benefits. It was a goal I had given myself.

Janet:	Does it help you cope?
Julie:	Yes, definitely.
Janet:	How does it help you cope?
Julie:	Um. I think to give yourself a task and get in and complete it is very important. My life has to revolve around goals, and part of that is being fit and healthy now. Also, it's probably the only time when I have any time to myself.

If a class was ever missed, mothers would express feelings of frustration, as Julie does here:

> Aerobic classes make me feel better about myself as a whole, as against the periods that I had been unable to attend that is, when I had some time off for the birth of my children. I felt much more frustrated if I was unable to get some form of exercise. Especially if I missed a class.

It is not necessary to remain always in a position of support in relation to power, as the women in these classes have demonstrated. The presence of resistance represents the possibility for change. The exercising women described how participation helped them cope with being a mum as it gave them a new feeling of freedom through accessing time for one's self:

- Gives me a break, puts my mind on other things.

- Because I can churn my energy into something else besides worry!! I feel that I am doing something for myself.

- To get away from home alone. Plus, I love to exercise. I feel better around people exercising.

- It's time for myself and I enjoy it.

- Because I am away from day to day housework.

When women exercise, it allows mothers to have a break and focus on something different. Exercise programs are effective in helping people to cope with stress because the people under stress are obliged to take time out from whatever they were doing and focus on something completely different. It could be the distraction and removal of the subject from the source of stress that is the effective mechanism, rather than aspects of the exercise process per se. This can be seen in a mother who has exercised and looks very relaxed, only to have a crying child thrust into her arms after the class and respond with tense facial expressions. A sense of coming back to reality and re-engagement with the usual role seem to take place. Time out may occur via a temporary mental distraction from stressors. This is most likely due to the change of physical location, the being engaged in movements to music and the change of mental focus and flow state that may result.

CONCLUSION

The consistent theme from the mothers' stories illustrated how through involvement in exercise for leisure, these women were able to resist any feelings of oppression or stress from the multiple roles of motherhood. The body, as a site for opportunities of disciplinary technologies, also offers opportunities to be a site for resistance to power. Foucault identified the body as a source of resistance. The body is never predictable or stable; it is elusive and capable of resistance within and outside of a discourse (Doering, 1992; Grosz, 1990; Looser, 1992; McWhorter, 1989):

> Moreover, particular discourses themselves offer more than one subject position. While a discourse will offer a preferred form of subjectivity, its very organization will imply other subject positions and the possibility of reversals (Weedon, 1987, p. 109).

Foucault calls on us to free the body and release it from the forces that hold it in their grasp. Mothers who take some time out for themselves are able to let go, even temporarily, of traditional roles and pressures which state that they should be 'on call' for other family members 24 hours a day. Through engagement in a reverse discourse, and taking time out to exercise, mothers may redefine their selfless roles. They also have an opportunity to lower their anxiety, raise their self-esteem and do something for themselves which is not always possible within the normal discourse of motherhood. 'We are never trapped by power, and it's always possible to modify its hold' (Foucault, 1980b, p. 13).

This is illustrated by the majority of participants believing that the classes reduced their stress levels and gave them a feeling of well-being, recuperation and time out for themselves. The positive benefits gained from resisting the motherhood role outweigh the argument that they may ironically work themselves harder afterwards. The women can still choose whether or not to overwork themselves, or whether they will delegate some tasks, develop time-management skills or have a rest break in the afternoon. The exercise classes may allow the mothers to feel better about housework or paid work because they've had some time for themselves.

The female body is the site of power that is, the locus of domination through which docility is accomplished and subjectivity constituted. This very focus of local and intimate operations of power (Foucault, 1977) can also be the site for resistance by women for creation of new space and time out. It has been shown through the qualitative data provided by the exercising women in this book that resistance through leisure provides a strategy for creation of one's own space, a feeling of freedom and well-being, and improved mental health. The reasons behind a mother being able to feel less stressed from participating in an exercise class may be described as:

1. having time out from multiple roles;

2. having a space of one's own, and

3. the distraction of the body moving through the exercise routine.

When mothers exercise for leisure, they can experience the freedom of doing something totally for themselves. Not for small children as a mother, or for an employer as a paid worker, but totally for themselves, by themselves. Exercise classes are also a break away from the notion that legitimate leisure for women is domiciled or home-based in nature. Foucault identified leisure as a form of male power (Rojek, 1985), and this is illustrated by the number of leisure facilities and recreational spaces which cater exclusively or largely for men, such as rugby league stadiums and cricket grounds. Social constraints are experienced disproportionately by women, especially women with children. The expectations associated with women's unpaid work impinge greatly on their available leisure time.

> Common denominators exist between the powerlessness that women find in their leisure and the powerlessness they find in other aspects of their lives (Henderson, 1990, p. 229).

The women's movement has been concerned with increasing the choice and entitlement of women. Mothers who attempt to add an extra role such as paid work to their existing load of being a career can end up with poorer mental health through task overload and role conflict. With increased numbers of mothers in paid employment, there has been little renegotiation of childcare and domestic duties, let alone allocation of leisure time in order for working mothers to recuperate from the extra burden (Losoncz, 2011). Women who reject traditional roles, who undertake exercise in their leisure time, who experience a space of their own, can feel less stressed as a result. However, women who have not yet tried exercise classes may not be aware of the benefits. Women are beginning to realise that time out for exercising is important for their own health, and that leisure offers a respite from the traditional caring role. As soon as there's a relation of power, there's a possibility of resistance (Foucault,1980b, p. 13).

The next chapter addresses some conflicting, less empowering aspects to exercise class participation.

Radical Leisure

CHAPTER 8

Disciplinary Effects of Exercise and the Body

INTRODUCTION

It has been shown in the previous two chapters how women may gain some relief from anxiety through exercising. However, women are exposed to great pressures from advertising, social media, and from the fitness industry itself, to conform to stereotypes about how they should look and behave (Maguire, 2008). Women can feel anxious about their bodies, and exercise may be seen as merely a vehicle to losing weight, rather than a means of coping with stress, or as something to be enjoyed.

Participating in exercise classes in a non-threatening, non-commercial setting reduces the stresses and strains of the motherhood role. Coming to the classes can be a form of time out and therefore a form of resistance to the socially acceptable roles of wife and mother. However, some of the participating mothers had a different story to tell about their motivations and the effects of the classes.

This chapter proposes that many women exercise to try to normalise their bodies and bring their body shape under control (similar to the aims of using a stomach control girdle). While it can be helpful to optimise our own body shape and tone, unfortunately many women feel pressured and attempt to use the classes as a means to lose weight. The normalisation processes described in this chapter are in contrast to the resistance discussion contained in Chapter 7. They include:

- women exercising to "normalise" the body and work towards the impossible ideal of being tall, thin, with a small waist, wide shoulders, narrow hips, flat stomach, tight bottom, and large breasts;

- mothers disciplining themselves to complete the classes or experiencing guilt as a result.

Some mothers expressed to me how they actively resisted the manipulations of popular media images and rejected the negative side of the discourse of fitness–exercise–figure improvement, which pressures and disciplines women to work out in order to more closely conform to the societal ideal. However, they were in the minority and I found that 94 per cent of my participants were attempting to tone their bodies or create an improved shape.

Disciplinary power is capable of creating docile bodies which attempt to conform to the social ideal through training or 'losing weight.' The pervasive awareness of the participants of the ideal body shape for women in general will now be discussed.

THE BODYWORKS ASPECTS OF THE EXERCISE CLASSES: THE DESIRE TO EXERCISE FOR SELF-IMPROVEMENT AND NORMALISATION OF BODY IMAGE

Joining the Classes to Lose Weight and Change Body Shape

Over 90 per cent of the women I surveyed for this book joined the exercise classes due to concerns about their body shape and image. These were typical reasons illustrating this point:

- I joined because, yes, I'm concerned with my body and wanted to exercise.

- Yes, I'm always trying to look better. Like I think I used to. Plus, to give me self-confidence.

- Yes, I mainly come to the classes to try to change my body shape and lose weight.

- I joined because, yes, I'm concerned with my body.

- Yes absolutely! To improve body shape.

- Yes, I mainly came to the classes to try to change my body shape and lose weight.

- Yes, I did come to the class in an effort to improve my figure and I started a diet on the same day I started the classes and I feel I have toned as well as lost a few kilos (7 kilograms).

Especially as weeks and months passed, the self-disciplining effect of the classes became even more important as many of the women expressed the wish to work on certain body areas, to lose fat from and improve certain parts of their bodies that they believed deviated from the society ideal. The mothers who had been relatively inactive since having a baby consistently endorsed this theme. As a sub-group, they were especially motivated by wanting to 'get back into shape,' as the following comments show:

- Need to get fit again and lose weight and tone up after just having second child.

- Wanting to get back into an exercise program and need to tone up and lose weight.

- Need to get in shape after having baby want to feel more energetic to keep up with baby!

- Need to get fit and lose some weight after having the children.

- Needing to tone up muscles all over. After having [the] second baby I've lost all my weight, but unfortunately have not exercised at all! (In 10 months).

- Need to regain fitness and lose weight I have not done very much since [having] children.

- I decided that it is time to ensure that I have a healthy lifestyle and I also know that I need to lose weight.

Amy explained that her motivation for taking part in the classes was to rid herself of post-baby weight gain:

- Helps me think that I'm trying to do something about getting rid of some of the extra weight that I put on through the baby.

For Janice, the body-trimming effects helped her feel happier, but there was still more work to do:

- I feel positive after the class with a brighter outlook on things. Also, when I see myself in my cosine I realise I have to keep going to try and improve my body shape. Tone the fat!

None of the women had been told by their doctors to lose weight. The urge or desire to lose weight had sprung up in their own minds. The majority revealed to me they had disciplined themselves to (a) join the exercise classes, and then (b) use the classes as a body shaping tool.

Belinda told me she did not join the class due to concerns with her body shape, "just for overall fitness, mental as well as physical." However, she then added, "being nearly 50, I feel I need more not less exercise as I get older, as your metabolism slows down and I love my food!" Therefore, she still wanted, like many of the other exercising mothers, to be in greater control of her body. Women build self-confidence through attaining the aesthetics of a thin and toned body (Markula, 1995):

The attractive female body has come to signify a controlled mind and healthy self-confidence (Markula & Pringle, 2006, p. 83).

What Does the Ideal Body Shape Look Like?

The women were also aware of the ideal body shape or image often portrayed in the media, which could pressure them to feel they had to look a certain way. When asked to describe this image, the responses consistently reflected themes of 'slim, young and beautiful':

- Big tits, very small waist, no stomach, tight bum, long legs. 20 years at 40!!

- Yes, I think the media portray the ideal woman as 16-18 years old, slim, sporty.

- You are always seeing beautiful, thin women in papers and magazines. Very rarely are the larger women portrayed. Ads on TV's are always slim, tanned, beautiful girls in bikinis. They try and use this concept to sell products.

- Yes, all the slim women in ads, never fat ones also young girls.

- Yes, the media is still promoting youthful, suntanned 16-18 year-old image sometimes too thin just so clothes look right in the magazine.

- Yes, they do. The body beautiful 'Elle' or similar. To be overweight is unhealthy.

- Yes, I think the media has a lot to do with women's figures.

- Like Elle McPherson for instance the image which for 99 per cent is an absolute impossibility.

- Slim, even SKINNY!!

- Sexy and slim.

- Women are always portrayed as sexy, beautiful models and with men lusting after them, tall, skinny, long hair, beautiful skin, tanned women who look mature about 25-29 years of age.

- Sun tanned Australian Iron-man type, or blonde, tall, athletic teenager girl.

- Tall, slender, good looking very fashionable.

- Media portrays an unreal trim, taut and terrific image, thus pressuring young women into eating disorders such as anorexia and bulimia in order to be accepted by peers and opposite sex.

- Barbie Doll images. Still with the tan even though they push block outs and 'stay out of the sun.' Most girls are over 5'6" tall.

However, Julie wished to qualify straight away that she did not agree with the ideal image often portrayed:

> [The media] makes you feel you should be ultra slim and beautiful. They forget about accepting your limitations and being a worthwhile person, who is fit and healthy, but [a] different shape.

Amy described the nature of the bulk of commercial fitness clubs as being dictated in terms of "competitive" dress norms and overrun with mirrors. She believed it would be difficult for most women, especially if overweight, to have the courage to enter many clubs due to self-consciousness:

> I think that there's a certain number of women out there well, as I said to you before wo not go to the gym. Um, they do not want to dress up in a leotard because they do not feel they have the body to compete against other people that do look nice in a leotard at the gym, and they like to just put on a pair of shorts and top and exercise in an atmosphere that's a lot more relaxed without feeling self-conscious. Because when you go to the gym, most of the people go there on a regular basis, and even if they're overweight like me at the moment, they're still really tight, their muscles still have some form to them.

SO, WHAT DOES A HEALTHY BODY SHAPE LOOK LIKE FOR A WOMAN?

The main themes arising from the women's descriptions of what a healthy body looked like for women included an emphasis on fitness, comfort, and health, in a kind of backlash to the very limiting images contained in fashion and the media:

- They should be portraying optimum health rather than body shape and size. Fitness and endurance rather than skinny versus fat. People should be the fittest and healthiest they can be for their natural body size and shape.

- What you feel comfortable with each to your own.

Secondly, most stated that a healthy body is a toned body, for example:

- I suppose a body looks healthy if it's well, and not flabby. It does not have to be muscly.

- There is no one right body shape; every person has different bone structures, height, etc. A healthy body shape is someone toned good muscle structure and who glows in the skin. Scale weight is not important the mirror is still the best judge.

- Taut body, clear smooth skin, shiny hair.

- Well-toned and trim.

The third theme in the description of healthy body shapes emphasised a well-proportioned body:

- In proportion. Not necessarily super thin. I prefer an athletic build to a fragile, narrow-shouldered build.

- Correct body weight and fit.

- I think a healthy body shape is [a] well-proportioned figure without looking too thin.

Yet, in this category, a few respondents actually specified what to them was a "healthy" measurement ideal, which actually mimicked a perfect hourglass figure:

- Women approximately 38"-28"-38". As long as you look and feel good that's the main thing.

- 36"-26"-36". Let's give them a chest and a little flesh. I do not want to see gaps between legs and not sticks for arms or legs or bones across chest.

How Does *Your* Body Look When It's at Its Healthiest?

There were only a few mothers taking part who felt that their bodies were at their healthiest at the moment, for example:

I am at my ideal weight now and nearly toned to my body/bone structure.

All but a few of the mothers participating in the classes wanted to lose some weight to feel "more comfortable" and therefore healthier:

- Would like to be, at this stage, thinner. I am working on it. However, I feel relatively fit, especially in view of having given birth 5+ months ago.

- The lower part of my body is overweight. If I were a stone lighter I know I would look better in clothes. Being overweight tends to make you a bit self-conscious when in bathing costumes or shorts.

- A comfortable size in clothes size 14. A size I know I can maintain.

- Lots of weight to lose, probably 40"-28"-40" would be OK I should probably work harder.

Some women believed their body would look its healthiest if they sculpted or reshaped particular parts of their body:

- For me my ideal would be first of all in the face pallor (healthy), strong shoulders, small waist, flat tummy, trim hips, strong slim legs, this is also my ideal shape for women generally.

- For me, I would prefer to be a bit taller, fuller breasted, slightly slimmer waist and tummy, and well-toned thighs and calves that fall straight from the hips.

- For me taller, smaller tighter bottom, smaller firmer hips.

The final category included a combination of losing weight, body part improvement and feeling fitter:

- I would like to have a flat stomach, be my correct weight (lose about one stone) and be able to perform energetic activities without effort.

- I think if I am within my weight for my height 50-55 kgs, and not too flabby, if I toned up. If I can handle a long brisk walk or an exercise class without too much strain then I would be more or less happy with my shape. 1 am trying to work towards this and with regular exercise and it seems to be working.

Therefore, sculpting certain areas or parts of the body was viewed as a way of feeling better about one's self. The desire for body normalisation could only be kept under control if the women had other objectives in mind, such as socialising or health-related concerns:

- Yes absolutely, I joined to improve body shape but also, I enjoy catching up with friends without children present.

- Firstly, to get rid of some anxiety and stress, then to feel better (mentally) in myself, then to be more aware of my body needs for toning up.

A fine line exists between the exercise helping women feel relaxed and better about themselves versus the women feeling they must attend classes as a means to control or correct defective areas.

How Does Exercise Help to Improve the Body Parts You Are Least Satisfied With?

The women felt that the exercise classes helped to improve the parts of the body causing them the most concern:

- Yes, I know the classes are helping these two parts as I feel tight the next couple of days later.

- Yes, especially the stomach. I feel the muscles are getting back to their old self after the birth of my baby.

- Yes, I feel the classes are working, combined with a diet I have lost 5 kg's and find that I have toned up a bit. I am feeling more fit.

- Yes, I can feel the exercise help because my body feels warm and stretched and itchy because I can feel the blood circulating.

- Yes, these exercises help all areas.

- Yes, my legs hurt so it must be working and hubby says I look better!!!

Some women felt that they still had "a lot more work" to do on rectifying certain body parts:

- This class has been good for all aspects may need a few more thigh exercises.

- I need a lot more work on my stomach, wish we had more stomach toning specifically.

- Yes, very much so. My stomach does not seem to be getting toned up. I have had 2 Caesars though, the 2nd being twins.

- Yes, it helps tone, but fat in these areas is difficult to move (Thighs, Stomach, Bottom).

The women tended to know they had improved the appearance of their body shape when they:

- received positive comments from others

- felt tightened and firmer muscles

- experienced weight loss

- had a flatter stomach

- perceived a better appearance in their own mind a feeling of greater satisfaction within themselves with areas of the body that normally caused concern or levels of dissatisfaction.

If exercise was deemed not to have helped with body shape improvement, this phenomenon was characterised by:

- muscles still slack, untoned, or flabby

- no weight loss having occurred

- the class not having focused on the particular problem areas of the body enough during the classes.

Many women expressed the need for the inclusion of more abdominal exercises. The stomach area was nominated as the body part that the respondents were least satisfied with (34 per cent), followed by thighs (23 per cent) and bottom (14 per cent).

SELF-DISCIPLINE INCREASES EXERCISE ADHERENCE

After 3 months, the reasons many of the mothers gave for still attending classes were self-discipline, motivation and having a routine. Sue explained that in order for her to attend, she needed "Just motivation, really, to get yourself there, and just keep going. That's really the secret." Other women said:

> I find it hard to find time to exercise, so this gives me a commitment to make sure I exercise.

> I think it started me on a routine of exercises. I had not been in them for a long time, and it sort of got me going regularly.

Karen thought that mothers would adhere to the program if they could make it part of a regular routine:

> It's just a matter of people getting into a routine, and you just organise it. Get going earlier.

With self-discipline cited by the women as a major factor which helped motivate them to attend the classes, this also led to an inner sense of guilt if they did not attend:

Oh yeah, you've done some exercise [laughs]. It's an achievement too when you have to go walking, you have to get yourself out of bed. Like it's real self-discipline. Aerobics I did because I knew, because, um. it's a discipline of there's a class and you know the time it's on and after a while if you do not go you start thinking, 'Well, I better not miss it,' because it's just a goal that you've put that's important, a priority, and if you do not go you feel guilty then, if you miss a class.

Attending classes can provide an inner sense of achievement. However, the routinisation, discipline, and organisation necessary to attend could be a source of stress in itself.

Disciplining the Body Toward a More Desirable Shape

We can develop an unhealthy link between our mind and body if we endlessly strive towards what we see as the socially desirable or beautiful. Markula and Pringle (2006, p. 80) proposed gym spaces and exercise practices as being designed to discipline our bodies towards "normalcy." However, we cannot achieve genuine stress reduction from exercise class participation unless we maintain a positive and realistic individual body image. If we perceive our body image through the eyes of others, we may be prone to this stress. For instance, an adolescent may be concerned with how others view their body. Women may be worried about how their body compares with society's ideal or norm, and whether their body shape or figure is considered attractive or unattractive as viewed through the eyes of others. It is not healthy to subordinate personal body image to assumptions of what others think of the body. This perspective entails the viewing of the body as if it were an object apart from oneself; for example, looking in the mirror and saying, "There's a fat slob" or "I wish those legs would get rid of their bulges." It is a process of objectifying body parts and depriving the body of its subjectivity.

The best possibility involves the person viewing her own body as self. The person accepts their whole body as is and says, "I am my body" (Marcel, 1952). This means that the person does not treat their body as compartmentalised and made up of parts, and is not worried about how it appears in other people's eyes. The person accepts and loves their whole body, with or without flaws.

However, I did hear negative comments from class participants that reflected poor attitudes towards various body parts, or the body as a whole. The disciplinary technology of the examination often involves influences from, and comparisons with, preconceived ideas, societal norms, fashions, media representations and images from advertisements. Through giving in to pressures from advertising, fitness ideologies and promotions (Maguire, 2008; Shaw & Kemeny, 1989), people are losing the power of direct control over their own bodies, as well as losing satisfied, self-controlled body perceptions. Their bodies are being used to achieve an outside goal, rather than their own.

People who are in the greatest psychological harmony with their physical bodies are considered the healthiest. Ironically, a certain amount of physical activity assists with positive body perception or image. There is also a strong connection between body image and self-esteem. A major barrier to the achievement of positive self-image and body perception is women's preoccupation with body weight and physical appearance.

It was evident from the research conducted for this book that the discourse of body image was an issue that all of the women were aware of. Body image refers to how an individual perceives one's physical self and includes surface, postural, and internalised pictures we have of our body as well as attitudes, emotions, and personality reactions. A certain amount of discipline is necessary in any exercise program, in order to adhere to the level of intensity and involvement necessary to reach basic health objectives such as cardiovascular benefits. When women discipline themselves within exercise programs at this pre-requisite level, they are most likely to achieve greater muscle toning, well-being, and an outlet for stress. They can be healthier, in greater control, raise their fitness and feel free to be involved in pleasurable activities. In this way, they work towards their own ideal body shape that is, the healthiest for their own bone structure, height, and body type. However, when women attempt to normalise their body shape towards the social ideal of a "supermodel," they then own "docile bodies" that are disciplined by the exercise in a more negative way.

Foucault (1977) described three technologies or ways in which power and knowledge are used to maintain the status quo: the examination, hierarchical observation, and normalising judgement. The body is a direct locus of social control through routines, rituals, practices, expectations, and certain actions. The discipline and normalisation of the female body has to be acknowledged as an amazingly durable and flexible strategy of social control (Bordo, 1992). Women are spending more time on the management and discipline of their bodies, producing docile bodies whose forces and energies are habituated to external regulation, subjection, transformation, and improvement (Bordo, 1992; Markula & Pringle, 2006).

Preoccupation with appearance still affects more women than men (Bordo, 1992). One effect of disciplinary power is that we can continue to "memorise on our bodies the feel and conviction of lack, insufficiency, of never being good enough" (Bordo, 1992, p. 14). In this way, the individual recognises and compares themselves in relation to normative discourses. A woman's dissatisfaction with her body will then result from the in-congruence of her perceived body size and shape with that which is culturally endorsed as ideal (van Gyn et al., 1989; Vannini & Waskul, 2006). The media and advertising have helped to create a world in which individuals are made to become emotionally vulnerable (Featherstone, 1982). This persuades them to adopt a critical attitude towards body, self and lifestyle (Sams & Keels, 2013). Therefore, self-examination can motivate the majority of women to attend, and keep attending, the classes, because they are critical of their body shapes and are attempting to improve them (Markula & Pringle, 2006).

Disciplinary technologies such as hierarchical observation, normalising judgement and the examination mean that individuals survey and discipline themselves in an attempt to maintain personal standards to an "acceptable" level. If a person fails to meet expected norms of behaviour, "little punishments" intended to make an example of the individual's failures are meted out (Doering, 1992, p. 29). Power is camouflaged, while compliance is reinforced. Routinisation and traditions in methods are expected, while deviations are not tolerated. There is an in-built need to discipline one's self to meet external expectations (Doering, 1992).

Therefore, a tension exists, because even though the women can have a break away from housework, some tend to:

1. attempt to complete more tasks when they arrive home in order to make up for time away from the housework schedule

2. routinise their exercise programs

3. discipline themselves to exercise to conform to the ideal body shape, or to lose weight, and

4. unwittingly or consciously feel a sense of commitment or obligation to conform to a healthier lifestyle by attending.

All of these factors can therefore reduce the sense of leisure and freedom the exercise class has the potential to bestow.

CONCLUSION

The aim of healthy exercise participation should be to reach your own optimal level of fitness, which is tied in with your own body shape. Regular exercise in moderation combined with a nutritious diet allows us to be closer to our own ideal for height, bone structure, body shape and genetics. We should feel better because we exercise, but not necessarily if we try, through exercise, to look like the stereotypical ideal. No amount of diet or exercise will give us that shape our ideal shape should be our own in its healthiest attainable form.

Some form of struggle, resistance or even conformity is always possible because the body is a site where power "inscribes itself, a modal point or nexus for relations of juridical and productive power" (Butler, 1989, p. 601). The classes do have a disciplining, self-surveillance side to them. This is in contradiction to the liberatory, freedom aspect of the classes. The positive aspects seem to out-weigh the negative; however, the women may be less conscious of the disciplinary power of the classes. According to Foucault's notion of "docile bodies," our bodies become amenable to normalisation through dominant discourses in our society, resulting in our exercising/practicing specific bodily movements to bring the body under control to conform to the specified requirements.

Exercise classes in a non-commercial setting have the capacity to reduce the stresses and strains of the motherhood role. Coming to classes is "time out" for some of them, and a form of resistance to the societally acceptable roles of wife and mother. However, a tension does seem to exist between the "ideal body image" motivation/result of exercising and the "something for myself" reason. The contradictions illustrate very well Foucault's notion of the body as a site of struggle, negotiations, resistances, and some possible transformations.

The mothers tended to discipline themselves to attend the classes in order to tone up, lose weight or have firmer muscles. Ironically, taking part in the exercise process does make them feel happier overall, because they:

1. feel as though they are taking positive steps towards improving their 'flawed' areas, which assists their body image/self-esteem,

2. feel fitter and healthier, which impinges positively on their mental outlook and sense of well-being.

When women participate in exercise classes, they can feel in greater control of the "destiny" of their body shape. However, in order to shape their bodies more closely to their own ideal, they have to discipline themselves to attend in order to strive for these goals. The classes therefore had a controlling effect over the women.

Therefore, the classes are both:

- self-examination

- self-surveillance

- disciplinary training

- normalising in relation to the body and to the expectations/discourses of good motherhood

and are:

- time out

- leisure

- liberating

- self-actualising, and

- resistance.

So, they are within the bounds of patriarchal or traditional power–knowledge–discourse, but are also resisting, pushing back the boundaries, allowing subjugated discourses to emerge and using the body to redefine subjectivity. The mothers are able to choose what the classes will mean to them, liberating or constraining. They do not have to dissect their bodies into parts and discipline themselves, even though they may feel pressure to do so. "Power is exercised only over free subjects, and only insofar as they are free" (Foucault, 1982b, p. 221). Mothers are faced with a range of possibilities in the ways they behave; they are not totally dominated by power, as this would equate to being a slave in chains (Foucault, 1982b). The mothers may have to engage in a struggle or feel stressed from rushing to attend the classes; however, the sense of freedom and stress relief that results is well worth the effort.

CHAPTER 9

Conclusion

EXERCISE CLASS PARTICIPATION: LIBERATION AND RELIEF?

This book has provided a unique insight into mothers' leisure experiences from a health-promoting perspective, outlining:

1. The reasons why mothers may wish to attend exercise classes and the individual benefits able to be attained;

2. Explanations for the sense of liberation and relaxation able to be achieved from the exercise experience, in women's own words;

3. The constraining nature of the body image discourse and use of exercise as a body sculpting tool by some mothers in order to improve areas viewed as deviating from the ideal.

The Lived Experience of Stress as Described by Mothers

The general nature of stress experienced by most mothers is a feeling of being trapped in a never-ending cycle of duties or schedule of activities that they discipline themselves to achieve:

> Everyday life, being a mother trying to get everything done and mainly getting irritable and tired.

> Just uptight and worrying about getting everything done that I want to get done, so that I can feel relaxed in myself.

This stress is caused by multiple roles or demands from various sources. Exercise has immense potential for relieving this stress in mothers. It helped all but two of the mothers I interviewed to "exercise their stress away." The reasons that the mothers provided for feeling less stressed after completing an exercise class included:

1. Time out from their assigned tasks and roles

2. A space of their own

3. The distraction process for example, the body moving through the exercise routine, coordinating the body to the music, and

4. Feeling the body gain muscle tone, fitness, and control.

The Contribution of Exercise Classes Toward Well-Being

Typical descriptions illustrating the positive potential of classes for enhancing a mother's subjective sense of well-being included:

- Well, once the music starts, and I get into the exercise, I just find that I am in a totally different, you know, [pause] space rather than at work, which you know is really good.

- Gives me a break, puts my mind on other things. The class alleviates these feelings of stress as I feel better able to cope mentally and physically.

- Relaxation, a feeling of well-being for you.

Exercise classes can also be a form of resistance for mothers. Women can let go of their motherhood role and escape, free from the normal compulsions associated with household duties. While they normally would not be able to switch off because of being constantly on the go, or caring for others, exercise enables mothers to find a new, separate space for themselves.

For the mothers I spoke to, getting involved in the classes can be difficult to achieve due to tiredness and stress experienced before the class. However, the body can always resist its situation; it is never totally trapped. It was therefore ironic to discover that many of the women were also involved in exercise classes in an attempt to try to improve their body shape and tone towards a slim ideal. The following responses characterise this phenomenon:

- I joined because, yes, I'm concerned with my body and wanted to exercise.

- Yes, I mainly come to the classes to try to change my body shape and lose weight.

- [Exercise] helps me think that I'm trying to do something about getting rid of some of the extra weight that I put on through the baby.

- Also, when I see myself in my cosine I realise I have to keep going to try and improve my body shape. Tone the fat!

Exercise classes can help to tighten stomach muscles, improve cardiovascular fitness and flexibility, and reduce the amount of "unhealthy flab." This can also help to raise self-esteem and mental well-being ("look good, feel good"). Fitness leaders and the broader health education of girls will need to be aware of the fine line between optimising body tone and shape and developing an unhealthy obsession. Many women in society use exercise as a perceived body-shaping tool. Power can discipline individuals into conforming, docile bodies. Unfortunately, the norm is for women to constantly, through cultural discourses, surveil themselves to make sure they are conforming to the normalised body image. Attempting to change one's body towards an external, impossible ideal is another form of achieving docility. Women need to set their own healthy goals, and only work towards optimising their own natural body shape, accepting its genetic limitations. Healthiest attitudes are those that include acceptance of the woman's own body and which resist pressures, expectations, or judgements from others. For example, Julie said that the media:

> makes you feel you should be ultra slim and beautiful. They forget about accepting your limitations and being a worthwhile person, who is fit and healthy, but [a] different shape.

Pauline also stated that:

> There is no one right body shape, every person has different bone structures, height, etc.

It is also healthy to have the amount of self-discipline necessary to adhere to the selected program. Finishing a class creates an inner sense of achievement. If the exercise process is sociable, fun, supportive, realistic, and enjoyable, then the habit of exercising will be made much easier to sustain.

Therefore, a paradox may exist between the self-surveillance and freedom aspects associated with exercise class participation. To a limited extent, exercise can help women feel like they are doing something to improve their appearance or the body parts that they are least satisfied with, and they can feel happier as a result.

RADICAL LEISURE: THE THEORETICAL AND HEALTH SIGNIFICANCE OF MOTHERS ACHIEVING TIME OUT

Exercise class participation is a means of gaining 'time out' for mothers. It can serve as a break from the normal routine, allowing for feelings of relaxation, rejuvenation, and revival. Taking time out to exercise can be thought of as the birth of a new, healthy lifestyle for stressed mothers. Leisure can be used as resistance to escape from entrapment in the home, or from tiring work regimes. In developing their own space, mothers can ease their stress levels and care for their own well-being. Mothers can develop strategies by themselves, with friends, or supported by community facilities and programs, in order to involve themselves in leisure activities and enjoy regular time out.

Throughout this book, Foucault's (1977) theory of power has been innovatively applied to health promotion (Table 9.1). Disciplinary technology constrains mothers; however, exercise classes provide a means of resistance to the stressful nature of the motherhood role. Individuals experience a greater sense of control over their own lives as a result:

> Feels good and I know it was for me my time.

> Basically, the first thing was doing something for me. After running around doing everything for the kids, I felt like I was actually doing something for me.

Table 9.1: A Comparison of the Main Theoretical Features of Health Promotion and Foucault.

Health Promotion	Foucault
• Helping people to gain control over the determinants of their own health. Leads to higher levels of subjective wellness. • A healthier body is more efficient and less likely to become sick. • Community participation, local self-determination, or control over the determinants of health. Self-responsibility and development of healthy knowledges, attitudes, and skills. • Healthy choices are 'good' choices; unhealthy choices are 'bad,' lazy, or unwise. • Lifestyle influences our health in the context of social and economic determinants. We have to overcome negative social - environmental impacts on our health. • Action and resistance carried out by individuals and development of healthy knowledge, skills, and attitudes. Higher levels of wellness are a prime objective. Wellness involves a dynamic process of responding to challenges and self-actualisation.	• Mothers resisting dominant motherhood discourse/other-centeredness and taking time out to exercise to reduce their stress. • Discipline intensifies the docility, capability, efficiency, and productivity of the body. • Possibility for resistance, active control in certain aspects of our life. Leisure as resistance. • Power can operate via the conscience and sense of morality. We discipline ourselves to be acceptable to society's norms. • We are always part of a network or forcefield of power relations. Power also exists in social relations. We have to often struggle to resist repressive disciplinary technologies to enable greater self-control. • Power transformation possible through struggles, resistance, and negotiations, which enables gain in well-being and greater control of situations.

Transformation at the conscious level means that freedom from the constraining ideology of body image discourse is possible. Power relations are not static or one-way. Power can gain or lose ground. Power also operates in small ways, which implies a better chance for transformation than if it were an all-dominating force. Without the possibility of recalcitrance, power would be the physical equivalent of a person in chains (Foucault, 1982b). The power of the ideologies surrounding motherhood mean that mothers unselfishly devote and submit themselves to home and family. Disciplinary technology restrains the mother in the home, maintaining the standard of care, cleaning, and housework. The silent hold over the docile body is to the benefit of others. Leisure works to free the body from this hold. Leisure resists the notion that housewives ought to be at home doing the housework and caring for the family 24 hours a day, not taking time out to play. The mothers' perceived benefits from class involvement relate to letting go of their normal selves and constraints:

> I can come here and forget who I really am and escape to another being, another person.

> [I gain] freedom on my own.

Leisure allows mothers to value themselves and challenges restrictions on individual freedom. It provides an opportunity for mothers to resist the normalising control of stereotyped motherhood ideologies. The original data accessed for this book has shown how the boundaries of home-bound mothers can be redefined and reconstructed. For many of the mothers in this book, leisure meant:

> Feeling like I am doing something for myself instead of staying home like a home-bound mother.

Researchers have recommended abandoning traditional gender role stereotypes as another way for women to gain time out:

> We all need to let go of the antiquated views of gender that see the female identity tied to caring and the male identity tied to winning bread. Both mums and dads are parents, and both are responsible for the care and well-being of their children. If the role of carer is more equally divided between both parents then it makes sense that working mums will have more time to look after themselves when they need it (Grace Papers, 2016).

We are never completely trapped by power. Points of resistance are present everywhere. Initial plans for change or recalcitrance can take place in the consciousness of the individual. For instance, the individual at a conscious level may think that she is "too fat," because she has sub-consciously measured and compared herself to societal standards such as magazine images or clothes sizes. However, at the conscious level she is able to challenge the negative self-talk and realise that self-acceptance of her own healthy body is best. Sub-conscious thoughts created through the disciplining effects of society's norms and pressures can be brought through to the conscious level and challenged, as in Figure 9.1.

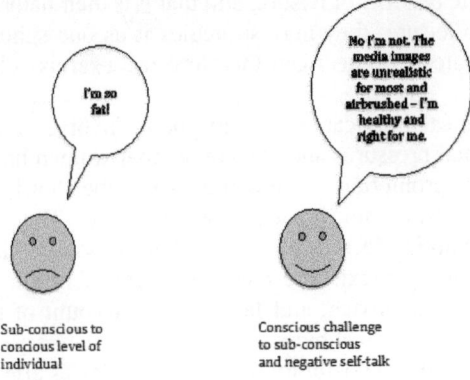

Figure 9.1: Initial Challenges Can Take Place at the Conscious Level of the Individual.

While leisure is an opportunity for women to resist the normalising, panoptic gaze of stereotyped motherhood ideologies, we must not 'blame the victim.' It's important to realise that there may be some mothers who are motivated and would love to take part, but who are single mothers constrained by their role, classes cost too much, or that there are other barriers to a woman's access to leisure. Being able to access leisure might not just involve a change of mindset. The *Strollers* Pram Walking program I devised is very successful, as it offers women an uncomplicated and free, easily accessible, and manageable form of physical activity that also removes the need for childcare (Currie & Develin, 1999, 2001; Develin & Currie, 2000).

Space is fundamental to resistance. The respondents explained how they could access time out and create a space for themselves. This concept is illustrated in Figure 9.2.

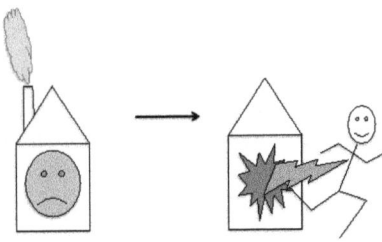

Figure 9.2: Taking Time Out to Escape the Feeling of Being Trapped at Home.

Once women realise the benefits of leisure, and that it is their natural right to regularly access and experience leisure, they may strategies it as one sphere where space for themselves can be created. Mothers can therefore use exercise classes to hold male power at bay.

The wider theoretical implications of this book involve recognising the many social and environmental pressures and constraints that women have to contend with. The focus of health promotion is moving from the level of individuals to organisations, communities, and broader social policy. The new public health approach to health promotion locates the etiology of disease within the occupational, social, and environmental context. The medical model of health seeks the cause of disease from a biological approach, and fails to take account of the social, political forces which can limit individual choices.

Health is an individual responsibility. Individual lifestyles affect individual health status. Individuals have to decide that they will exercise because no one else can do it for them. A certain amount of self-discipline is needed to be able to adhere to the exercise program. The mothers contributing their stories to this book recommended approaches to help make it work:

> It's just a matter of people getting into a routine, and you just organise it. Get going earlier.

> Just motivation, really, to get yourself there, and just keep doing. That's really the secret.

Health promotion programs also have to take into account, however, that not everyone has an equal capacity to choose certain lifestyle behaviours, due to barriers or constraints. Some women may feel too depressed or unsafe to exercise. Structural constraints limiting mothers' opportunities for participation include:

- socioeconomic discrimination, or cost prohibition, especially for single mothers

- inappropriate and inadequate media coverage

- lack of suitable or conveniently located programs that provide appropriate class time schedules, exercise intensities, a friendly, safe atmosphere, or accommodation for childcare

- lack of time available due to current work and family arrangements; and

- lack of exercise partners.

Ideological constraints arise from the traditional characteristics and expectations associated with the motherhood role. The ethic of care suggests that it is the responsibility of mothers to place others' needs first. Ideological and social factors which may also limit mothers' participation in exercise include:

- feeling responsible for domestic duties

- lack of self-confidence or feelings of self-worth or entitlement

- not feeling "sporty" or young enough to suit the activity

- feeling too fat, unfit, or non-conforming with the slim, ideal standards existing in many commercial, mirror-walled settings.

Therefore, health professionals are faced with a dilemma in policy-making. Unless the individual takes some responsibility, it is impossible for them to enter the wellness/wholeness state. However, this needs to be balanced with recognition of the structural impediments. Moral approaches to health promotion are intolerant of the barriers and constraints existing in society, and this may ironically lead to an unethical "blame the victim" policy. We need to identify ways to break down the constraints.

In response to the above issues, practical strategies which may work towards facilitating an individual's commitment and involvement in exercise include:

- utilising a 'bottom-up' approach to community program development which focuses on the needs and wants of local mothers;

- providing free child-minding facilities;

- ensuring programs are held in convenient, safe locations;

- providing special classes for beginners, the very unfit, pregnant or overweight;

- allowing and promoting a wider optional range of clothing than is considered suitable to wear to exercise classes;

- improving the people skills of gymnasium staff and including wider age groups in selected staff so that fitness centres are more accepting, welcoming and user-friendly;

- promoting the acceptance of various individual female body shapes in exercise programs and description of them in neutral terms;

- providing a safe, 'embarrassment-free' exercising environment with private changing cubicles, if required;

- placing a greater emphasis on the fun and social aspects of the exercise process;

- ensuring a manageable intensity level in exercise classes for mothers which (a) allows for mingling and conversation before, during and after the class, (b) is not high-impact, and (c) involves emphasis on strengthening abdominals, legs, chest and back, plus improvement of cardiovascular fitness;

- educating instructors and participants to not regard or promote exercise as a ready means to drastically alter the shape of particular body parts;

- regulating inappropriate advertising that attempts to intertwine health or exercise with unrealistic sex, beauty, or youth messages;

- providing positive physical education experiences at school which enhance the prospect of women wishing to engage in physical activity as a lifelong pursuit;

- allowing mothers discounted or concessional program rates, subsidised by the federal health and/or sports departments, in order to improve participation;

- developing a promotional campaign encouraging mothers to take part in community exercise classes which provides positive role models and helps to allay guilt feelings, while promoting friendship, relaxation and enjoyment.

THE IMPLICATIONS FOR PUBLIC POLICY

The creation of supportive environments will do much to assist mothers in their quest for leisure: "Work and leisure should be a source of health for people" (WHO, 1986, p. 2). For the mothers who are involved in outside work, a health break during the day or walking during lunchtime may be the only chance they have of obtaining time out to exercise or relax. There needs to be increased access for mothers to participate in council-run leisure facilities and exercise programs.

Building healthy public policy means that health is placed on the agenda of all policy-makers in all sectors and at all levels. Sport has continued to become more commercialised, business-like, and professional in all aspects. Increasing participation in sport and sport activities by all Australians requires that access to sporting activities has to be thought of more as a community health, welfare and recreational strategy for all, not just for the sporting elite.

Most people will make decisions to act (health behaviours and choices), from the range of options available to them (opportunities for making choices). Mothers will most likely choose the least costly option in deciding whether to exercise or not. This will involve evaluating factors such as costs related to dollars, time and availability of childcare, compared with the perceived benefits and value associated with the activity. All healthy decisions are affected by socioeconomic circumstances and ease of choice. Therefore, any policies guiding practical initiatives in physical activity promotion for mothers may take the following factors into account:

1. Appropriateness and Convenience of Setting:

The least travel time, expenditure and disruption involved to other activities, the more likely that mothers will engage in physical activity. Exercise sites for mothers who work primarily at home need to be within easy walking distance or have free car parking. Conveniently located, pleasant settings assist mothers pushing strollers or caring for young children. The mothers in this book who primarily completed work inside the home felt that the most convenient time is mid-morning, immediately after they have dropped their children at school. If the time is too late, then the mothers can feel that they do not have enough time left to complete any outstanding housework and other tasks.

Selecting existing community facilities such as playgroups, schools, community centres and church halls may help the mothers to feel more relaxed and comfortable; like they 'own' the space. This may facilitate interaction amongst the group before and after the class. There also is not another class waiting to use the previous class' space.

Mothers involved in work outside the home will benefit from provision of change and shower facilities at work. Exercise breaks or classes provided for staff can take place in existing meeting or canteen areas if no gym is available.

2. Setting Realistic and Appropriate Targets:

Some physical activity is better than none. Fifty per cent of people who start exercise programs drop–out within 6 months. Part of the reasons may be because they set targets that were unrealistic or the class intensity was too high. There needs to be greater availability of 'lite pace,' low impact and lower intensity classes for mothers.

Even though the benefits of incidental physical activity such as stair climbing or hanging the washing out are promoted as legitimate exercise in the fight against heart disease, they are not as conducive to stress reduction in mothers if the mother is simultaneously climbing the stairs with two toddlers, a pram and shopping bags; or the physical tasks such as washing or vacuuming are always conducted by the mother and are considered by her to be 'work,' not active leisure.

3. Media, Marketing, & Promotions:

The media can be seen as key strategy for the advancement of women. Media is a powerful influence in people's lives. Presentation of positive role models and a variety of realistic body shapes at all levels throughout the media will contribute to the long-term commitment to gender equity in leisure. Mothers would like to see a more representative and realistic portrayal of themselves to illustrate their diversity in age, ethnic background, body shape, work and family roles and various aspirations.

If the value of the activity is highlighted in promotions, mothers will be more likely to be attracted to, and persist, with the program. The emphasis in a marketing approach is on determining the customer's needs and wants and then fulfilling these needs. The mothers in this program were asked why they joined in order to ascertain their needs, goals and reasons for attending. It became clear that concerns with improving body shape and muscle tone were most important to the mothers and gave meaning and motivation to program attendance.

Marketing of exercise needs to emphasise a variety of body shapes and mothers who have improved their health status. The mental and social benefits of exercise are also relevant to marketing plans. Stress relief and time away from busy work schedules are benefits that can be highlighted to mothers who are thinking about whether to exercise or not.

4. Specificity:

The more specific the aim of an exercise promotion campaign or message, the more likely it is to be successful. The exercising mothers in this book felt more confident about attending because they could relate to the other women, and were from similar backgrounds and circumstances.

The specific benefits need to be tailored to each group. Program managers need to talk to each group to find out their needs and wants and understand their requirements. The respondents enjoyed the benefits of childcare, time and freedom for self, and the chance to meet other local mothers.

5. Social Networks:

Mothers drawn from the exercise group may be most effective in influencing their peers to exercise. Utilising word-of-mouth and existing mothers' networks such as school parents' groups or early childhood centres, will reach a wide audience. Mothers could also be recruited by state health and sports agencies to be trained as exercise class leaders.

6. **Advice and Assistance:**

The mental health benefits of exercise classes for mothers may be promoted to GPs. Inactive mothers often ask medical or health professionals for advice on how to take up exercise. Inactive mothers as well as mothers who are already active who would like to exercise more, would also like the opportunity to exercise with others. For safety and social reasons, community messages and meeting points need to be promoted for mothers to be able to meet and exercise in groups. Community messages advertising fitness classes can be posted in pharmacy windows, shops, doctor's surgeries and social media networks.

THE FUTURE

This book provides some of the first in-depth validations in Australia of the benefits that mothers can gain from exercise class participation; they can feel better afterwards and enhance their mental well-being. However, mothers can enjoy the benefits that exercise has to offer if they choose to participate or resist the constraints that may be present.

To understand mothers' leisure, a holistic approach is helpful to acknowledge the complexities and structural impediments existing in their lives. That is, the mothers' leisure experiences described in this book need to be situated within a broader societal context, taking into account socioeconomic factors, gender, education levels and various other social and agency constraints such as:

- the increasing number of mothers engaging in full-time employment;

- the unchanging sexual division of labour in the home;

- increasing fears, anxiety and risks associated with violence in society;

- the lack of female leisure spaces, appropriate programs and childcare facilities available to women as mothers;

- the high costs of participating in commercial leisure for women (who make up the majority of low-income earners and sole parents); and

- mass media images which stereotype or limit women's aspirations.

While we cannot ignore the repressive nature of structural constraints on women in society, it is possible (in Australia) for individual action and shifts of power at the micro level. Mothers who access exercise classes are not passive and compliant; they choose to liberate themselves from traditional subjectivities, even if gaining only temporary respite:

- I felt young again, free again, forgot everyday life.

- It's time away to think about myself.

- It's a reward. It's something for yourself. And it's for you, whereas it's not for anyone else, you know, cause you're a mother, and you're a wife, and an auntie this is just for you.

A wider implication of this book relates to the social and environmental determinants of health status that is, the effect of the mass media on women's conscious or unconscious beliefs about body image. The mental health and stress reduction benefits gained from participating in exercise to music classes can be emphasised, rather than pressuring women to attempt to achieve an 'ideal' body shape (Currie, 2004, 1994). Greater research is needed on the specific benefits to women's body image, self-esteem and mental health from exercise programs which focus on optimising women's own potential body shape and fitness, within their own realistic limits and genetic determinations.

In stating that exercise programs can reduce stress in working mothers, this book is proposing a non-medical answer or response to the problem. Health promotion is able to challenge the medicalisation of health, which relies on an ideology that blames each person. Biomedical approaches individualise health problems, rather than recognising the social circumstances and determinants of health (Palmer & Short, 1994). As most of the participants expressed a fear of entering a commercial gym, but not of attending a local community hall class (solely for women), the intimidatory factors surrounding the fitness industry obviously need to be addressed (Currie, 1994). As this woman explained:

I think that there's a certain number of women out there, well as I said to you before, would not go to the gym, um, they do not want to dress up in a leotard because they do not feel they have the body to compete and they like to exercise in an atmosphere that's a lot more relaxed without feeling self-conscious.

Fitness clubs must defy and counteract cultural and body image stereotypes in the way their classes are delivered.

CONCLUSION: FEELING A DIFFERENCE

Mothers who engage in exercise classes to music may gain mental well-being and easing of stress levels. This book has demonstrated that mothers who make the commitment to take time out to exercise feel 'a difference' in their lives, in that they:

- feel more relaxed and in control

- feel less frustrated and worried

- are more optimistic

- have improved coping ability.

It has also provided enlightenment at the micro level of the meaning of this leisure experience for mothers, within a health and lifestyle context. At the macro level, society has not developed the attitude that exercise is a normal, legitimate and health-promoting right for mothers working primarily inside and/or outside the home, over their other responsibilities. We have to broaden the availability of exercise classes to a wider range of women in the community, for example through council recreation programs, to enable greater numbers of mothers to benefit. Otherwise, as Amy concluded, 'women who have not done it before might not know the difference' that exercise can make to a mother's health and mental fitness.

While policy-makers cannot ignore the structural constraints to women's health and leisure, class, gender and practical constraints are not completely deterministic. Even when policies remove some of the financial, geographical or ideological barriers, individuals must nevertheless make an active choice. Supportive environments and healthy policies that take into account the lifestyles of mothers will ensure that individual action towards leisure is facilitated.

Mothers can passively accept current lifestyle patterns and social relations, or they can actively seek out new directions for themselves, confronting the challenges. The body is a site of struggle. At the individual level, negotiations, motivations, and resistances can lead to transformation of power relations and ultimately greater opportunities for mothers' health and leisure. Exercise classes provide a definite avenue for mothers to promote their mental well-being. The mothers in this book are also in a better position to be able to materialise their leisure opportunities and overcome challenges, because the classes left them with greater self-confidence and feelings of control.

While the settings of everyday life could be more conducive and supportive to women's health promotion, women need to resist in order to carve out the necessary space and time that they need in their daily schedules for leisure. Leisure can be a source of self-nurturance recuperation, relaxation, and renewal, if the desire for this space or time out is materialised via strategies of negotiation, resistance, or recognition of self-worth. Policies in wider society can facilitate access to such personal spaces for all women, and for mothers in particular, and are in need of careful consideration and planning by policy-makers in the health area. The demands on women working at home and/or in the workforce will not decrease into the 2020s. Strategies that enable women to take more control of their own lives and deal with the stressors imposed upon them cannot be ignored.

REFERENCES

Abood, D. (1984). The Effects of Acute Physical Exercise on the State Anxiety and Mental Performance of College Women. *American Corrective Therapy Journal, 38*(3), 69–74.

Allen, M. E. (1990). Endorphin's Role as a Mood Modifier. *Annals of Sports Medicine, 5*(2), 89–95.

American Psychological Association. (APA). (2011). *Parenting: Being supermom stressing you out?* Accessed from www.apa.org/helpcenter/supermom.aspx

Anderson, E., & Shivakumar, G. (2013). Effects of Exercise and Physical Activity on Anxiety. *Frontiers in Psychiatry, 4,* 27, 1–4.

Anshel, M. (2006). *Applied Exercise Psychology A practitioner's guide to improved client health and fitness.* NY: Springer.

Anthony, J. (1991). Psychologic Aspects of Exercise. *Clinics in Sports Medicine, 10*(1), 171–180.

Australian Bureau of Statistics (ABS). (2015). *4177.0 Participation in Sport and Physical Recreation, Australia, 2013–14.* Accessed from http://www.abs.gov.au/ausstats/abs@.nsf/mf/4177.0

Australian Bureau of Statistics (ABS). (2013a). *4156.0.55.001* Perspectives on Sport, June 2013. *Women in Sport: The State of Play 2013.* Accessed from http://www.abs.gov.au/ausstats/abs@.nsf/Products/4156.0.55.001~June+201 3~Main+Features~Women+in+Sport+The+State+of+Play+2013?OpenDocu ment

Australian Bureau of Statistics (ABS). (2013b). *4364.0.55.004 Australian Health Survey: Physical Activity, 2011–12.* Accessed from http://www.abs.gov.au/ausstats/abs@.nsf/Lookup/4364.0.55.004main+featur es12011-12

Australian Bureau of Statistics (ABS). (2012a). *Mother's Day 2012: More mums heading to work. Media Release, 8 May 2012.* Accessed from http://www.abs.gov.au/ausstats/abs@.nsf/Lookup/by per cent20Subject/4125.0~Jan per cent202012~Media per cent20Release~Mother's per cent20Day per cent202012: per cent20More per cent20mums per cent20heading per cent20to per cent20work per cent20(Media per cent20Release)~6153

Australian Bureau of Statistics (ABS). (2012b), *4364.0.55.001 Australian Health Survey: First results.* Canberra: Australian Bureau of Statistics.

Australian Bureau of Statistics (ABS). (2012c). *4177.0 Participation in Sport and Physical Recreation, Australia, 2011–12.* Accessed from http://www.abs.gov.au/ausstats/abs@.nsf/Previousproducts/4177.0Main per cent20Features32011-12?opendocument&tabname=Summary&prodno=4177.0&issue=2011-12&num=&view=

Australian Bureau of Statistics (ABS). (2009). *4102.0 Australian Social Trends, Trends in Household Work.* Accessed from http://www.abs.gov.au/AUSSTATS/abs@.nsf/DetailsPage/4102.0March per cent202009?OpenDocument

Australian Bureau of Statistics (ABS). (2008). *4326.0 National Survey of Mental Health and Wellbeing: Summary of Results, 2007, Australia.* Accessed from http://www.ausstats.abs.gov.au/ausstats/subscriber.nsf/0/6AE6DA447F985F C2CA2574EA00122BD6/$File/43260_2007.pdf

Australian Department of Health & Ageing. (ADHA). (2005). *Women's Health Australia. The Australian Longitudinal Study on Women's Health. Research Highlights The first decade.* Canberra: ADHA.

Australian Government Department of Health (AGDH). (2014). *Australia's Physical Activity and Sedentary Behaviour Guidelines. Guidelines Evidence Summary.* Accessed from http://www.health.gov.au/internet/ main/publishing.nsf/Content/3768EA4DC0BF11D0CA257BF0001ED77E/$ File/Guideline per cent20Evidence per cent20Summary.PDF

Australian Psychological Society (APS). (2015). *Stress and Wellbeing. How Australians Are Coping with Life. The Findings of the Australian Psychological Society Stress and Wellbeing in Australia Survey 2015.* Accessed from https://www.psychology.org.au/Assets/Files/PW15-SR.pdf

Bahrke, M. S., & Morgan, W. P. (1978). Anxiety Reduction Following Exercise and Meditation. *Cognitive Therapy Research, 2,* 323–333.

Barsky, A. J. (1988). *Worried Sick: Our troubled quest for wellness.* Boston: Little, Brown.

Bartky, S. (1988). Foucault, Femininity and the Modernization of Patriarchal Power. In I. Diamond & L. Quinby. (Eds.), *Feminism and Foucault: Reflections on Resistance* (pp. 61–86). Boston: Northeastern University Press.

Baxter, J. (2013). *Families working together. Getting the balance right.* Canberra: Australian Institute of Family Studies, Australian Government.

Beggs, S., Vos, T., Barker, B., Stevenson, C., Stanley, S., & Lopez, A. D. (2007). *The burden of disease and injury in Australia, 2003.* Canberra: Australian Institute of Health and Welfare.

Ben-Tovim, D. (1992). All the Flavour and None of the Guilt. In Fact or Fiction? Dieting, Body Image and Women's Health, National Conference Proceedings (pp. 4–16). Saturday, 11 July 1992, Sydney.

Berger, B. G. (1984a). Running Strategies for Women and Men. In M. L. Sachs & G.W. Buffone. (Eds.). *Running as Therapy: An integrated approach* (pp. 23–62). Lincoln: University of Nebraska Press.

Berger, B. G. (1984b). Running Away from Anxiety and Depression: A Female as Well as Male Race. In M. L. Sachs & G.W. Buffone. (Eds.). *Running as Therapy: An integrated approach* (pp. 138–171). Lincoln: University of Nebraska Press.

Berger, B. G. (1984c). Running Toward Psychological Well-Being: Specific Considerations for the Female Client. In M. L. Sachs & G.W. Buffone. (Eds.). *Running as Therapy: An integrated approach* (pp. 172–197). Lincoln: University of Nebraska Press.

Berger, B. G., & Owen, D. R. (1989). Mood Alteration in Yoga and Swimming: Aerobic Exercise Not Necessary. Paper presented at the North American Society for the Psychology of Sport and Physical Activity, Annual Meeting. Kent State University, USA, 1-4 June.

beyondblue. (2016). *Pregnancy and Early Parenthood. Emotional Health.* Accessed from https://www.beyondblue.org.au/who-does-it-affect/pregnancy-and-early-parenthood/emotional-health

Biddle, S. (1991). *Psychology of Physical Activity and Exercise.* NY: Springer-Verlag.

Biddle, S. (1995). "Exercise and Psychological Health." *Research Quarterly for Exercise and Sport, 66,* 292–297.

Biddle, S., Fox, K. R., & Boutcher, S. H. (Eds.). (2000). *Physical Activity and Psychological Well-Being.* London: Routledge.

Biddle, S., & Mutrie, N. (2007). *Psychology of Physical Activity: Determinants and Well-Being.* (2nd ed.). Hoboken, NJ: Taylor & Francis.

Biddulph, J., Elliot, K., Faldt, J., Fowler, P., & Dugdale, A. (1984). The Body Image and Health-Related Behaviour of Teenage Girls. *Journal of Food and Nutrition, 41*(1), 33–36.

Black, J., Chesher, G. B., & Starmer, G. A. (1979). The Painlessness of the Long-Distance Runner. *Medical Journal of Australia, 1,* 522–523.

Blair, S. N., Kohl, H. W., & Barlow, C. E. (1993). Physical fitness and all-cause mortality: A prospective study of healthy men and women. *Journal of the American College of Nutrition, 12,* 368–371.

Bordo, S. R. (1992). The Body and the Reproduction of Femininity: A Feminist Appropriation of Foucault. In A. M. Jaggar & S. R. Bordo (Eds.), *Gender/Body/Knowledge: Feminist reconstructions of being and knowing* (pp. 13-33). Piscataway, NJ: Rutgers University Press.

Botkin, D. (1989). Coping with the Dual Career Marriage. *Medical Aspects of Human Sexuality. Feb:* 66–79.

Bouchard, C., & Johnson, F. E. (1988). *Fat Distribution During Growth and Later Health Outcomes.* NY: Alan Liss.

Brown, H., Abbott, G., Pirotta, S., & Camilleri, R. (2017). *Jean Hailes Women's Health Survey 2017. Understanding health information needs and health behaviour in women in Australia.* Accessed from https://jeanhailes.org.au/contents/documents/News/2017_WHW_Annual_survey_report_2017.pdf.

Brown, J. D. (1991). Staying Fit and Staying Well. *Journal of Personality, Sociology and Psychology, 60*(4), 555–561.

Brownell, K. D. (1991). Dieting and the Search for the Perfect Body: Where Physiology and Culture Collide. *Behavior Therapy, 22,* 1–12.

Bull, F. C., Bauman, A. E., Bellew, B., & Brown, W. (2004). *Getting Australia Active II: An update of evidence on physical activity for health.* Melbourne, Australia: National Public Health Partnership (NPHP).

Butler, J. (1989). Foucault and the Paradox of Bodily Inscriptions. *Journal of Philosophy, 86*(11), 601–607.

Byrne, A., & Byrne, D. (1993). The Effects of Exercise on Depression, Anxiety and Other Mood States: A Review. *Journal of Psychosomatic Research, 37*(6), 565–574.

Carmack, M. A., & Martens, R. (1979). Measuring Commitment to Running: A Survey of Runners' Attitudes and Mental Status. *Journal of Sport and Psychology, 1,* 25–42.

Carpenter, G., & Sheklow, S. (1985). The Leisure–Feminism Link. *Leisure Information Quarterly, 2*(3), 5–6.

Carr, D., Bullen, B., Skinar, G., Arnold, M., Rosenblatt, M., Beitins, I., Martin, J., & McArthur, J. (1981). Physical Conditioning Facilitates the Exercise-Induced Secretion of B-endorphin and B-lipotropin in Women. *New England Journal of Medicine, 302*, 560–563.

Cash, T. F., Novy, P. L., & Grant, J. R. (1994). Why Do Women Exercise? Factor Analysis and Further Validation of the Reasons for Exercise Inventory. *Perceptual and Motor Skills, 78*, 539–544.

Cenovis. (2017). *Because We Know You Do not Always Put Yourself First.* Accessed from cenovis.com.au/women.

Chernin, K. (1993). *Womansize: The tyranny of slenderness.* NY: Harper and Row.

Choi, P. Y. L., Van Horn, J. D., Picker, D. E., & Roberts, H. I. (1993). Mood Changes in Women after an Aerobics Class: A Preliminary Study. *Health Care for Women International, 14*, 167–177.

Clow, A., & Edmonds, S. (2014). *Physical Activity and Mental Health.* Champaign, IL: Human Kinetics.

Cohn, L. D., Adler, N. E., Irwin, C. W., Millstein, S. G., Kegeles, S.M., & Stone, G. (1987). Body Figure Preferences in Male and Female Adolescents. *Journal of Abnormal Psychology, 96*(3), 276–279.

Cooke, K. (1994). *Real Gorgeous. The truth about body and beauty.* Sydney: Allen & Unwin.

Coovert, D. L., Thompson, J. K., & Kinder, B. N. (1988). Interrelationships among Multiple Aspects of Body Image and Eating Disturbance. *International Journal of Eating Disorders, 7*, 495–502.

Cox, R. (2013). *Sport Psychology: Concepts and applications.* (7th ed.). NY: McGraw-Hill.

Cramer, S. R., Nieman, D. C., & Lee, J. W. (1991). The Effects of Moderate Exercise Training on Psychological Well-being and Mood State in Women. *Journal of Psychosomatic Research, 35*, 437–449.

Csikszentmihalyi, M. (1975). *Beyond Boredom and Anxiety.* San Francisco: Jossey-Bass.

Csikszentmihalyi, M., & Csikszentmihalyi, I. (1988). *Optimal Experience: Psychological studies of flow in consciousness.* NY: Cambridge University Press.

Csikszentmihalyi, M., & Kleiber, D. (1991). Leisure and Self-Actualization. In B. L. Driver, P.J. Brown & G. Peterson. (Eds). *Benefits of Leisure* (pp. 91–102). State College, PA: Venture Publishing.

Currie, J. L. (2009) Managing Motherhood: Strategies Used by New Mothers to Maintain Perceptions of Wellness. *Health Care for Women International, 30*(7), 653–668.

Currie, J. L. (2004). Motherhood, Stress, and the Exercise Experience: Freedom or Constraint? *Leisure Studies, 23,* 225–242.

Currie, J. L. (1994). Fit and Fashionable Body Images: Are They Alienating the Female Fitness Industry Market? In *Towards 2000: Proceedings of the NSW ACHPER Conference* (pp. 1–6). 22–24 September 1994, Sydney University.

Currie, J. L., & Develin, E. D. (2001). Stroll Your Way to Well-Being: A Survey of the Perceived Benefits, Barriers, Community Support, and Stigma Associated with Pram Walking Groups Designed for New Mothers. *Health Care for Women International, 23*(8), 882–93.

Currie, J. L., & Develin, E. D. (1999). *Stroll Your Way to Well-Being. A guide to the planning and organization of pramwalking groups in order to increase the mental health of mothers and decrease the risk of postnatal depression.* Wolloomooloo, NSW: NSW Government Department of Women.

Davidson, P. (1992). Contributions of a Holiday to Women's Lives. In Recreation and Wellness: National Recreation and Wellness Conference Proceedings, 12–13 March 1992, Phillip Institute of Technology, pp. 105–116.

Davis, C. (1990). Body Image and Weight Pre-Occupation: A Comparison between Exercising and Non-Exercising Women. *Appetite, 15*(1), 13–21.

Davis, L. L. (1985). Perceived Somatotype, Body Cathexis and Attitudes toward Clothing Among College Females. *Perceptual and Motor Skills, 61,* 1190–1205.

Dawson, D. (1988). The Rational Subordination of Women's Leisure under Patriarchal Capitalism. *Society and Leisure, 11*(2), 397–411.

De Benedette, V. (1988). Getting Fit for Life: Can Exercise Reduce Stress? *Physician and Sports Medicine, 16*(6), 185–200.

De Geus, E. J. C., Van Doomen, L. J. P., & Orlebeke, J. F. (1993). Regular Exercise and Aerobic Fitness in Relation to Psychological Make-up and Physiological Stress Reactivity. *Psychosomatic Medicine, 55,* 347–363.

De Vaus, D. (2009). Balancing Family Work and Paid Work: Gender-based Equality in the New Democratic Family. *Journal of Family Studies, 15*(2), 118–121.

Deem, R. (1986). *All Work and No Play.* Milton Keynes, UK: Open University Press.

Deem, R. (1982). Women, Leisure and Inequality. *Leisure Studies, 1*(1), 29–46.

Develin, E. D., & Currie, J. L. (2000). The Strollers Pramwalking Program: A Community Intervention Aimed at Increasing the Physical Activity Level of Mothers with Young Children. *Health Promotion Journal of Australia, 10*(1), 57–59.

Diamond, I., & Quinby, L. (1988). Introduction. In I. Diamond & L. Quinby. (Eds.), *Feminism and Foucault. Reflections on resistance* (pp. ix-xx). Boston: Northeastern University Press.

Dienstbier, R. A., Crabbe, J., Johnson, G. O., Thorland, W., Jorgensen, J. A., Sadar, M. M., & La Velle, D. C. (1981). Exercise and Stress Tolerance. In M. H. Sacks & M. L. Sachs (Eds.), *Psychology of Running* (pp. 192–210). Champaign, Illinois: Human Kinetics.

Dinucci, J. M., Finkenberg, M. E., McCune, S. L., McCune, E. D., & Mayo, T. (1994). Analysis of Body Esteem of Female College Athletes. *Perceptual and Motor Skills, 78*, 315–319.

Doering, L. (1992). Power and Knowledge in Nursing: A Feminist Poststructuralist View. *Advances in Nursing Science, 14*(4), 24–33.

Dorinsky, N. (1984). Brief Reports: The Effects of a Regular Aerobic Exercise Program on Selected Measures of the Stress Response. *Health Care for Women International, 5*, 459–462.

Dove. (2017). *Our Research.* Accessed from http://www.dove.com/us/en/stories/about-dove/our-research.html.

Dove. (2016). *The Dove Global Beauty and Confidence Report. New Dove Research Finds Beauty Pressures Up, and Women and Girls Calling for Change.* Accessed from http://www.prnewswire.com/news-releases/new-dove-research-finds-beauty-pressures-up-and-women-and-girls-calling-for-change-583743391.html.

Dreyfus, H., & Rabinow, P. (1982). *Michel Foucault: Beyond structuralism and hermeneutics.* Chicago: Harvester Press Ltd.

Driscoll, R. (1976). Anxiety Reduction Using Physical Exertion and Positive Images. *Psychological Record, 26*, 87–94.

Driver, B. L., Brown, P. J., & Peterson, G. L. (1991). *Benefits of Leisure.* State College, PA: Venture Publishing.

Duquin, M. E. (1989). Fashion and Fitness: Images in Women's Magazine Advertisements. *Arena Review, 13*(2), 97–109.

Dworkin, S. L. (2009). *Body Panic, Gender, Health, and the Selling of Fitness.* NY: New York University Press.

Farrell, P. A. (1985). Exercise and Endorphins: Male Responses. *Medicine and Science in Sports and Exercise, 17*(1), 89–93.

Farrell, P. A., Gates, W., Maksud, M., & Morgan, W. (1982). Increases in Plasma B-endorphin/B-lipotropin Immuno-reactivity after Treadmill Running in Humans. *Journal of Applied Physiology, 52,* 1245–1249.

Featherstone, M. (1982). The Body in Consumer Culture. *Theory, Culture, and Society, 1*(2), 18–33.

Foucault, M. (1988). On Power. Interview by Pierre Boncenne with Michel Foucault. In L. Kritzman. (Ed.). *Michel Foucault: Politics, Philosophy, Culture. Interviews and Other Writings 1977-1984* (pp. 96-109). (Translated by Sheridan, A.). NY: Routledge.

Foucault, M. (1987). The Ethic of Care for the Self as a Practice of Freedom. In J. Bernauer & D. Rasmussen. (Eds.), *The Final Foucault* (pp. 1–20). Cambridge, MA.: Massachusetts Institute of Technology Press.

Foucault, M. (1982a). Space, Knowledge and Power Interview with Michel Foucault. In P. Rabinow. (Ed.). (1984), *The Foucault Reader* (pp. 239–256). NY: Pantheon Books.

Foucault, M. (1982b). The subject and power. In H. L. Dreyfus & P. Rabinow. (Eds.), *Michel Foucault: Beyond Structuralism and Hermeneutics* (pp. 208–226). Brighton, UK: Harvester Press.

Foucault, M. (1980a). The History of Sexuality, Vol 1. (Translated by Hurley, R.). NY: Pantheon Books.

Foucault, M. (1980b). The History of Sexuality: An Interview. (Translated by Bennington, G.). *Oxford Literacy Review, 4*(2), 13.

Foucault, M. (1979a). Powers and Strategies. In M. Morris & P. Patton. (Eds.), *Michel Foucault: Power, Truth, Strategy* (pp. 49–58). Sydney: Feral Publications.

Foucault, M. (1979b). Power and Norm: Notes. In M. Morris & P. Patton. (Eds.), *Michel Foucault: Power, Truth, Strategy* (pp. 59–66). Sydney: Feral Publications.

Foucault, M. (1977). *Discipline and Punish.* (Translated by Sheridan, A.). London: Penguin Books.

Foucault, M. (1976). Two Lectures. In C. Gordon. (Ed.), *Michel Foucault. Power/Knowledge: Selected Interviews and Other Writings 1972–1977* (pp. 78–108). NY: Harvester Press.

Frazier, S., & Nagy, S. (1989). Mood State Changes of Women as a Function of Regular Aerobic Exercise. *Perceptual and Motor Skills, 68*(1), 283–287.

Gellhorn, S. (2016). *Postnatal Depression and Maternal Health: A handbook for frontline caregivers working with women with perinatal mental health difficulties.* Hove, UK: Pavilion.

Gjerdingen, D., McGovern, P., Bekker, M., Lundberg, U., & Willemson, T. (2000). Women's Work Roles and Their Impact on Health, Well-being, and Career: Comparisons between the United States, Sweden and the Netherlands. *Women and Health, 31,* 1–17.

Glassner, B. (1988). *Bodies: Why we look the way we do and how we feel about it.* NY: Putnam.

Goldfarb, A. H., Hatfield, D., Sforzo, F. A., & Flynn, G. (1987). Serum B-endorphin Levels during a Graded Exercise Test to Exhaustion. *Medicine and Science in Sports and Exercise, 19,* 78–82.

Grace Papers (2016). *Mums working longer hours than CEOs.* Accessed from https://gracepapers.com.au/mums-working-longer-hours-than-ceos/.

Grossman, A., & Sutton, J. R. (1985). Endorphins: What Are They? How Are They Measured? What Is Their Role in Exercise? *Medicine and Science in Sports and Exercise, 17*(1), 74–81.

Grosz, E. (1994). *Volatile Bodies: Toward a corporeal feminism.* Sydney: Allen & Unwin.

Grosz, E. (1991). *Rethinking the Body.* Presentation at Body Politics. Women's Studies Centre Seminar, University of Sydney, NSW, Australia. 19 October 1991.

Grosz, E. (1990). Contemporary Theories of Power and Subjectivity. In S. Gunew. (Ed.), *Feminist Knowledge: Critique and Construct* (pp. 59–120). London: Routledge.

Haier, R. J., Quaid, K., & Mills, J. S. C. (1981). Naloxone Alters Pain Perception after Jogging. *Psychiatric Research, 5,* 231–232.

Hamilton-Smith, E., & Driscoll, K. (1990). *Measuring the Benefits of Recreation.* Bundoora, Victoria: Department of Leisure Studies, Phillip Institute of Technology.

Harber, V. J., & Sutton, J. R. (1984). Endorphins and Exercise. *Sports Medicine, 1*(2), 154–171.

Hart, E. A., Leary, M. R., & Rejeski, W. J. (1989). The Measurement of Social Physique Anxiety. *Journal of Sport and Exercise Psychology, 11*, 94–104.

Harvey, J., & Sparks, R. (1991). The Politics of the Body in the Context of Modernity. *Quest, 43*, 164–189.

Henderson, K. (1990). The Meaning of Leisure for Women: An Integrative Review of the Research. *Journal of Leisure Research, 22*(3), 228–243.

Henderson, K. A., Bialeschki, M. D., Shaw, S. M., & Freysinger, V. J. (1989). *A Leisure of One's Own. A feminist perspective on women's leisure.* Philadelphia, US: Venture Publishing.

Hitchcock, K. (2009). *Little White Slips.* Sydney: Pan Macmillan.

Hochschild, A. (1989). *The Second Shift.* NY: Penguin Books.

Hogan, C. (1995). The incredible shrinking woman. *Good Weekend,* March, 44-51.

Holden, L., Dobson, A., Byles, J., Chojenta, C., Dolja-Gore, X., Harris, M., Hockey, R., Lee, C., Loxton, D., McLaughlin, D., Mishra, G., Pachana, N., Reilly, N., & Tooth, L. (2013). *Mental Health: Findings from the Australian longitudinal study on women's health. May 2013.* Canberra: Australian Government Department of Health and Ageing.

Howson, A. (2004). *The Body in Sociology.* Cambridge: Policy Press and Blackwell.

Hull, R. B. (1991). Mood as a Product of Leisure: Causes and Consequence. In B. L. Driver, P.J. Brown, & G. Peterson. (Eds.), *Benefits of Leisure* (pp. 249–262). State College, PA: Venture Publishing.

Huon, G. (1992). Psychological Aspects of Dieting and Body Image among Adolescents and Young Women. In *Fact or Fiction? Dieting, Body Image and Women's Health, Proceedings of a National Conference.* 11 July 1992, Sydney, pp. 19–27.

Huon, G.F., Morris, S.E. & Brown, L.M. (1990). Differences between male and female preferences for female body size. *Australian Psychologist, 2*(3), 314–317.

Imm, P. & Pruitt, J. (1991). Body Shape Satisfaction in Female Exercisers and Non Exercisers. *Women and Health, 17*(4), 87–96.

Imm, P. (1990). Perceived Benefits of Participants in an Employees Aerobic Program. *Perceptual and Motor Skills, 71*(3), 753–754.

Iwasaki, Y., Mannell, R., Smale, B., & Butcher, J. (2005). Contributions of Leisure Participation in Predicting Stress Coping and Health among Police and Emergency Response Services Workers. *Journal of Health Psychiatry, 10*(1), 79–99.

Kagan, E., & Morse, M. (1988). The Body Electronic. Aerobic Exercise on Video: Women's Search for Empowerment and Self-Transformation. *Drama Review, 32,* 164–180.

Kelly, D. D. (1986). *Stress Induced Analgesia.* NY: Academy of Science.

Kelson, T. R., Kearney-Cooke, A., & Lansky, L. M. (1990). Body Image and Body Beautification Among Female College Students. *Perceptual and Motor Skills, 71,* 281– 289.

Kenen, R. (1987). Double Messages, Double Images: Physical Fitness, SelfConcepts and Women's Exercise Classes. *Journal of Physical Education, Recreation and Dance, 58*(6), 74–79.

Kolb, L. (1959). Disturbances of Body Image. In G. van Gyn, J. Raddulph & R. Bell (Eds.). (1989). *Proceedings of the Jyvaskyla Congress on Movement and Sport in Women's Life* (pp. 465–476). 17–21 August, Jyvaskyla, Finland. Vol 1.

Krejci, R., Sargent, R., Forand, K., Ureda, J., Saunders, R., & Durstine, J. (1992). Psychological and Behavioural Differences Among Females Classified as Bulimic, Obligatory Exerciser and Normal Control. *Psychiatry, 55,* 185–193.

Labbe, E., Welsh, M., & Delaney, A. (1988). Effects of Consistent Aerobic Exercise on the Psychological Functioning of Women. *Perceptual and Motor Skills, 65*(3), 919–925.

Lam, L., & Riba, M. (2016). *Physical Exercise Interventions for Mental Health.* Cambridge, UK: Cambridge University Press.

Lazarus, R. (1980). The Stress and Coping Paradigm. In C. Eisdorfer, D. Cohen, A. Kleinman, & P. Maxim. (Eds.) (pp. 177–214). *Theoretical Bases for Psychopathology.* NY: Spectrum.

Lee, C. (2001). Family Caregiving: A Gender-Based Analysis on Women's Experiences. *Australian Institute of Family Studies Published Papers, 68,* 123–139.

Leith, L., & Taylor, A. (1990). Psychological Aspects of Exercise: A Decade Review. *Journal of Sport Behaviour, 13*(4), 219–239.

Lemert, C. C., & Gillan, G. (1982). *Michel Foucault: Social Theory and Transgression.* NY: Columbia University Press.

Lenskyj, H. (1988). Measured Time: Women, Sport and Leisure. *Leisure Studies, 7*(3), 233–240.

Lenskyj, H. (1991). The Leisure/Pleasure Connection in Women's Lives. *Paper presented at the World Congress, World Leisure and Recreation Association.* 16–19 July, Sydney, Australia.

Long, B., & Haney, C. (1988a). Coping Strategies for Working Women: Aerobic Exercise and Relaxation Interventions. *Behaviour Therapy, 19,* 75–83.

Long, B., & Haney. C. (1988b). Long-Term Follow-up of Stressed Working Women: A Comparison of Aerobic Exercise and Progressive Relaxation. *Journal of Sport and Exercise Psychology, 10,* 461–470.

Long, B.C. (1983). Aerobic Conditioning and Stress Reduction: Participation or Conditioning? *Human Movement Science, 2*(3), 171–186.

Looser, D. (1992). Feminist Theory and Foucault: A Bibliographic Essay. *Style, 26*(4), 593–603.

Losoncz, I. (2011). Persistent Work–Family Strain among Australian Mothers. *Family Matters, 86,* 79–88.

Maguire, J. (2008). *Fit for Consumption: Sociology and the business of fitness.* NY: Routledge.

Marcel, G. (1952). *Metaphysical Journal. Translated by Bernard Wall.* Chicago, US: Henry Regnery.

Markoff, R. A., Ryan, P., & Young, T. (1982). Endorphins and Mood Changes in Long-Distance Running. *Medicine and Science in Sports and Exercise, 14,* 11–15.

Markula, P. (1995). Firm but Shapely, Fit but Sexy, Strong but Thin': The Postmodern Aerobicizing Female Bodies. *Sociology of Sport Journal,* 15, 109–37.

Markula, P. & Pringle, R. (2006). *Foucault, Sport and Exercise: Power, knowledge and transforming self.* London: Routledge.

Martinson, E. W., Hoffart, A., & Solberg, O. Y. (1989). Aerobic and Non-Aerobic Forms of Exercise in the Treatment of Anxiety Disorders. *Stress Medicine, 5*(2), 115–120.

McWhorter, L. (1989). Culture or Nature? The Function of the Term 'Body' in the Work of Michel Foucault. *Journal of Philosophy, 86*(11), 608–614.

Morgan, W. P. (1985). Affective Beneficence of Vigorous Physical Activity. *Medicine and Science in Sports and Exercise, 17*(1), 94–100.

Morgan, W. P. (1979). Anxiety Reduction Following Acute Physical Activity. *Psychiatric Annals, 9*, 36–45.

Morgan, W. P., Horstman, D. H., Cymerman, A., & Stokes, J. (1980). Exercise as Relaxation Technique. *Primary Cardiology, 6*, 48–57.

Niven, C. & Carroll, D. (1993). *The Health Psychology of Women.* Sydney: Harwood Academic Publishers.

Noles, S. W., Cash, T. F., & Winstead, B. A. (1985). Body Image, Physical Attractiveness, and Depression. *Journal of Consulting and Clinical Psychology, 53*, 88–94.

NSW Consultative Committee (NSWCC). *If Motherhood Is Bliss, Why Do I Feel So Awful?' Community consultations on postnatal stress and depression in NSW.* Woolloomooloo: NSW Department for Women.

O'Dea, J. (2007). *Everybody's Different: A positive approach to teaching about health, puberty, body image, nutrition, self-esteem and obesity prevention.* Camberwell, Vic.: ACER Press.

O'Dea, J. (1992). Poor Body Image and Women What Are the Adverse Effects? In *Fact or Fiction? Dieting, Body Image and Women's Health. Proceedings of a National Conference.* 11 July 1992, Sydney, pp. 29–40.

Orbach, S. (1985). *Fat Is a Feminist Issue.* London: Hamlyn.

Padawer, W. J. & Levine, F. M. (1992). "Exercise-Induced Analgesia: Fact or Artifact?." *Pain, 48*, 131–135.

Palmer, G.R. & Short, S.D. (1994). *Health Care and Public Policy.* South Melbourne: Macmillan.

Paluska, S., & Schwenk T. (2000). Physical Activity and Mental Health: Current Concepts. *Sports Medicine, 29*(3), 167–80.

Pargman, D. & Baker, M. C. (1980). Running High: Enkephalin Indicted. *Journal of Drug Issues, 3*, 341–350.

Patton, P. (1979). Of Power and Prisons. In M. Morris & P. Patton. (Eds.). *Michel Foucault: Power, Truth, Strategy* (pp. 109–147). Sydney: Feral Publications.

Patty, A. (2016). Working mothers put their health second, research shows. *The Sydney Morning Herald, May 10.* Accessed from http://www.smh.com.au/business/workplace-relations/working-mothers-put-their-health-second-research-shows-20160510-goqk09.html

Paxton, S. J., Werthein, E. H., Gibbons, K., Szmukler, G. I., Hillier, L., & Petrovich, J.L. (1991). Body Image Satisfaction, Dieting Beliefs and Weight Loss Behaviours in Adolescent Boys and Girls. *Journal of Youth and Adolescence, 20*(3), 361–379.

Payne L. (2010). Relations between Leisure, Health, and Wellness. In L. Payne L, B. Ainsworth & G. Godbey. (Eds.). *Leisure, Health, and Wellness: Making the connections* (pp. 21–29). State College, PA: Venture Publisher.

Pearce, J. (1993). Women's Bodies, Women's Exercise. *Australian Journal of Leisure and Recreation, 3*(2), 39–44.

Pearce, J. (1989). *Supermum Survival Hints for Working Mothers. Report of a Women's Health Forum.* Mona Vale, NSW: Mona Vale Hospital Health Promotion Unit.

Perutz, K. (1970). *Beyond the Looking Glass: Life in the beauty culture.* London: Hodder & Stoughton.

Rabinow, P. (1984). *The Foucault Reader.* Middlesex, England: Penguin.

Racevskis, K. (1993). Interpreting Foucault. *Papers on Language and Literature, 29,* 96–110.

Reavely, N. J., Jorm, A. F., Cventovski, S., & MacKinnon, A. J. (2011). "National Depression and Anxiety Indices for Australia. *Australian and New Zealand Journal of Psychiatry, 45,* 780–787.

Redican, B. & Hadley, D. (1988). A Field Studies Project in a City Health and Leisure Club. *Sociology of Sport Journal, 5,* 50–62.

Richins, M. (1991). Social Comparison and Idealized Images in Advertising. *Journal of Consumer Research, 18,* 71–83.

Rojek, C. (1985). *Capitalism and Leisure Theory.* London: Tavistock Publications, Inc.

Rosato, F. D. (1990). *Fitness and Wellness: The Physical Connection.* St. Paul, MN: West Publishing Company.

Roth, D. L. (1989). Acute Emotional and Psycho-physiological Effects of Aerobic Exercise. *Psychophysiology, 26*(5), 593–602.

Sachs, M. (1982). Running Therapy: Change Agent in Anxiety and Stress Management. *Journal of Health, Physical Education, Recreation and Dance, 53*(7), 44–45.

Saltman, D. (1991). *Women and Health.* Sydney: Harcourt Brace Jovanovich.

Salusso-Deonier, C. J., Markee, N. L., & Pedersen, E. L. (1993). Gender Differences in the Evaluation of Physical Attractiveness Ideals for Male and Female Body Builds. *Perceptual and Motor Skills, 76,* 1155–1167.

Sanford, W. (1984). Body Image. In The Boston Women's Health Book Collective. (Ed.). *The New Our Bodies, Ourselves* (pp. 5–10). NY: Simon & Schuster, Inc.

Sams, L. B., & Keels, J. A. (2013). *Handbook on Body Image.* NY: Nova Publishers Inc.

Saunders, K. (1994). Why women tear themselves to bits. *She,* September, 66–67, 143.

Sawicki, J. (1991). *Disciplining Foucault: Feminism, power and the body.* NY: Routledge.

Schafer, W. (1987). *Stress Management for Wellness.* Florida, USA: Holt, Rinehart & Winston.

Schulte, B. (2014). *Overwhelmed: Work, love, and play when no one has the time.* London: Bloomsbury.

Schulze, L. (1990). On the muscle. In J. Gaines & C. Herzog. (Eds.). *Fabrications: Costume and the female body* (pp. 59–78). NY: Routledge.

Seyle, H. (1974). *Stress Without Distress.* NY: Harper & Row.

Shank, J.W. (1986). An Exploration of Leisure in the Lives of Dual Career Women. *Journal of Leisure Research, 18*(4), 300–319.

Shaw, S., & Kemeny, L. (1989). Fitness Promotion for Adolescent Girls: The Impact and Effectiveness of Promotional Material Which Emphasizes the Slim Ideal. *Adolescence, 24*(95), 677–687.

Silberstein, L., Striegel-Moore, R., Timko, C., & Rodin, J. (1988). Behavioural and Psychological Implications of Body Dissatisfaction: Do Men and Women Differ? *Sex Roles, 19*(3/4), 219–231.

Simons, A. D., McGowan, C. R., Epstein, L. H., Kupfer, D. J., & Robertson, R. J. (1985). Exercise as a treatment for depression: An update. *Clinical Psychology Review, 5,* 553–568.

Slade, T., Johnston, A., Teeson, M., Whiteford, H., Burgess, P., Pirkis, J., & Saw, S. (2009). *The Mental Health of Australians 2: Report on the 2007 National Survey of Mental Health and Wellbeing.* Canberra: Commonwealth Department of Health and Ageing.

Smith, J. (1995). *'Women Tearing Ourselves Apart': A Study of Women's Attitudes Towards Their Thighs.* Unpublished BHMS (Hons.) Thesis. North Sydney: Australian Catholic University.

Smyth, M. (1991). *Balancing Acts: Managing home and work.* Sydney: NSW Women's Advisory Council.

Spielberger, C. D. (1989). Stress and Anxiety in Sports. In D. Hackfort & C. D. Spielberger. (Eds.). *Anxiety in Sports: An international perspective* (pp. 3–7). Washington, USA: Hemisphere.

Steel, A., Frawley, J., Dobson, A., Jackson, C., Lucke, J., Tooth, L., Brown, W., Byles, J., & Mishra, G. (2013). *Women's Health in NSW A life course approach: An Evidence Check rapid review brokered by the Sax Institute.* Sydney: Sax Institute.

Steinberg, H., & Sykes, E. A. (1985). Introduction to Sympos-ium on Endorphins and Behavioural Processes; Review of Literature on Endorphins and Exercise. *Pharmacology, Biochemistry and Behaviour, 23,* 857–862.

Swan, N. (2006). *Postnatal Depression.* Canberra, ACT: Rural Health Education Foundation.

Taylor, C., Sallis, J., & Needle, R. (1985). The Relation of Physical Activity and Exercise to Mental Health. *Public Health Reports, 100*(2), 195–202.

Theberge, N. (1991). Reflections on the Body in the Sociology of Sport. *Quest, 43,* 123–134.

Theberge, N. (1987). Sport and Women's Empowerment. *Women's Studies International Forum, 10,* 387–393.

Thompson, J. K. (1990). *Body Image Disturbance: Assessment and treatment.* NY: Pergamon.

Tiggemann, M., & Pennington, B. (1990). The Development of Gender Differences in Body Size Dissatisfaction. *Australian Psychologist, 2*(3), 306–313.

Tiggemann, M. & Rothblum, E. (1985). A Cross-Cultural Study of Attitudes to Weight. In E. Kerby-Eaton & J. Davis. (Eds). *Women's Health in a Changing Society: 2nd National Conference on Women's Health.* SACAE, Magill Campus. pp. 142–147.

Travis, C.B. (1988). *Women and Health Psychology.* New Jersey: Lawrence Earlbaum Associates Inc.

Treble, G., Blacklock, F., & McCormack, W. (1990). Self-Image and Body Composition in Females. In *27th National Annual Scientific Conference*

Proceedings, Australian Sports Medicine Federation Limited. 11–13 October, Alice Springs, NT. pp. 76–90.

Tucker, L.A. (1985). Dimensionality and Factor Satisfaction of the Body Image Construct: A Gender Comparison. *Sex Roles, 12,* 931.

van Gyn, G., Randolph, J., & Bell, R. (1989). Body Image of Active Women as Related to Age. In *Proceedings of the Jyvaskyla Congress on Movement and Sport in Women's Life.* 17–21 August 1987, Jyvaskyla, Finland, Vol 1, pp. 465–475.

van Minnen, A., Hendriks, L., & Olff, M. (2010). When Do Trauma Experts Choose Exposure Therapy for PTSD Patients? A Controlled Study of Therapist and Patient Factors. *Behavioral Research Therapy, 48,* 312–20.

Vannini, P., & Waskul, D. (2006). *Body/embodiment: Symbolic interaction and the sociology of the body.* Alder-shot, Hants, UK: Ashgate.

Vargas, R. (2015). *Body Image: Social influences, ethnic differences and impact on self-esteem.* Hauppauge, NY: Nova Science.

Wankel, L. M. (1992). The Social Psychology of Physical Activity an Active Living Perspective. In *Recreation and Wellness, National Recreation and Wellness Conference Proceedings.* 12–13 March 1992, Phillip Institute of Technology, pp. 173–213.

Wankel, L. M., & Berger, B. (1990). The Psychological and Social Benefits of Sport and Physical Activity. *Journal of Leisure, 22,* 167–182.

Warrick, R. & Tinning, R. (1989). Women's Bodies, Self-Perception, and Physical Activity: A Naturalistic Study of Women's Participation in Aerobics Classes, Part 1. *The ACHPER National Journal, 125,* 8–12.

Wearing, B. (1998). *Leisure and Feminist Theory.* London: Sage.

Wearing, B. (1990). Beyond the Ideology of Motherhood: Leisure as Resistance. *Australian and New Zealand Journal of Sociology, 26*(1), 36–58.

Wearing, B. (1989). Leisure, Unpaid Labour, Lifestyles and the Mental and General Health of Suburban Mothers. *Australian Journal of Sex, Marriage, and Family, 10*(3), 118–132.

Wearing, B. (1984). *The Ideology of Motherhood.* Sydney: Allen & Unwin.

Wearing, B. & Wearing, S. (1990). Leisure for All? Gender and Policy. In D. Rowe & G. Lawrence. (Eds.). *Sport and Leisure: Trends in Australian Popular Culture* (pp. 161–173). Sydney: Harcourt Brace Jovanovich.

Wearing, B., & Wearing, S. (1988). All in a Day's Leisure: Gender and the Concept of Leisure. *Leisure Studies, 7,* 111–123.

Weedon, C. (1987). *Feminist Practice and Poststructuralist Theory.* Oxford: Basil Blackwell.

Weinberg, R., Jackson, A., & Kolodny, K. (1988). The Relationship of Massage and Exercise to Mood Enhancement. *Sports Psychologist, 2*(3), 202–211.

Weiss, P. (1979). The Challenge of the Body. In E. W. Gerber & W. J. Morgan. (Eds.). *Sport and the Body: A philosophical symposium* (pp. 188–191). Philadelphia: Lea & Febiger.

WHO/FIMS Committee on Physical Activity for Health. (1995). Update/Le Point: Exercise for Health. *Bulletin of the World Health Organization, 73*(2), 135–136.

Wilfley, D. E., Grilo, C. M., and Brownell, K. D. (1994). Exercise and Regulation of Body Weight. In M. M. Shangold & G. Mirkin. (Eds). *Women and Exercise: Physiology and sports medicine.* (2nd ed.) (pp. 27–54). Philadelphia: F.A. Davis Company.

Williamson, K. (1981). The tyranny of slimness. *National Times,* November, 19–21.

Wimbush, E. (1986). *Women. Leisure and Well-Being.* Edinburgh: Centre for Leisure Research.

Wolf, N. (1994). *The Beauty Myth.* London: Vintage.

Woods, N. (1980). Women's Roles and Illness Episodes: A Prospective Study. *Research in Nursing and Health, 3*(4), 134–145.

Woolhouse, H., Gartland, D., Mensah, F., & Brown, S. J. (2014). Maternal depression from early pregnancy to 4 years postpartum in a prospective pregnancy cohort study: implications for primary health care. *British Journal of Obstetrics & Gynaecology, 122*(3), 312–321.

World Health Organization (WHO). (2016). *Physical Inactivity: A Global Public Health Problem. Global Strategy on Diet, Physical Activity, and Health.* Accessed from http://www.who.int/dietphysicalactivity/factsheet_inactivity/en/

World Health Organization (WHO). (2009). *Global health risks: mortality and burden of disease attributable to selected major risks.* Accessed from http://www.who.int/healthinfo/global_burden_disease/GlobalHealthRisks_report_full.pdf

World Health Organization (WHO). (1986). *Ottawa Charter for Health Promotion.* Geneva: World Health Organ-isation.

Young, R.J. (1979). The Effect of Exercise on Cognitive Functioning and Personality. *British Journal of Sports Medicine, 13,* 110–117.

INDEX